Praise for *Play Hard, Di*

"Dr. Omalu's book should frighten every football player in America. His autopsies of NFL stars are persuasive evidence that the game has produced tens of thousands of brain injuries. He argues with great good sense that the epidemic can be traced to a macho culture in which players, coaches, officials, parents, and even physicians turn a blind eye to football's obvious dangers. This book can be the beginning of change that enriches the game and saves lives."

—**Dave Kindred**
*Best-selling author and winner of the Red Smith Award
for lifetime achievement in sports journalism*

"The long-time elephant in the NFL's kingdom is finally exposed in *Play Hard, Die Young*, a disturbing book that will make you think twice the next time one of your Sunday heroes makes a crunching tackle or gets pounded by a helmet to the jaw as he fights for extra yards. This ought to be must-reading for every player, coach, trainer, and team doctor in the league, as well as the owners who pay them to risk limb and life every time they take the field, but never seem to worry about the truth regarding traumatic head injuries and their terrible short and long-term consequences."

—**Leonard Shapiro**
Washington Post

"As someone who loves the NFL and profits from it, reading this book made me uncomfortable. But it is an important book that needs to be read—especially by parents who are considering letting their sons play football and by anyone who plays football, as well as their loved ones."

—**Dan Pompei**
Chicago Tribune

"Mind-boggling. This thought-provoking book portrays a revealing look at the dark side of football, and Dr. Omalu should be commended for addressing such a sensitive subject, one that affects thousands of young men who play the game."

—**Ralph Wimbish**
New York Post

"Dr. Omalu offers a chilling and disturbing account of the dark side of our beloved yet violent game. This is an interesting and required read for anyone who wears a football helmet and bangs his head for a living or even for recreation. Just his detail alone on Mike Webster, Andre Waters, and Terry Long will make you understand the dangers of concussions and the threat of dementia . . . it's a very interesting book that comes at the right time, what with scores of retired players suffering from one game-related malady or another."

—Shaun Powell
Newsday

"We've come a long way . . . but as Bennet Omalu's book, *Play Hard, Die Young*, tells us, there's still a ton of room for improvement. As technology improves in the coming years, especially in the helmet, we may eventually look back at a Mike Webster the way we look at early auto racers who died due to the lack of safety equipment we consider standard today."

—**Ken Willis**
The News-Journal (Daytona Beach, FL)

"An eye-opening read for football fans. Players past and present—and young, aspiring players, too—need this information. It could wind up saving their lives."

—**Bob D'Angelo**
The Tampa Tribune

"You aren't likely to see *Play Hard, Die Young* advertised on NFL.com. Dr. Omalu's book is a clear, concise, compassionate study of the delayed brain damage that is suffered by pro football players as a result of repeated concussions. If most of us are unfamiliar with the term "gridiron dementia," it's because the NFL and mainstream media have done a good job of underreporting and minimizing concussions. Dr. Omalu shines a bright light on a subject that deserves more attention."

—**Bob Molinaro**
The Virginian-Pilot (Norfolk, VA)

PLAY HARD, DIE YOUNG

.

PLAY HARD, DIE YOUNG

Football Dementia, Depression, and Death

BENNET OMALU, MD

Neo-Forenxis^{SM} **Books**

LODI, CALIFORNIA

Neo-Forenxis Books
1132 Junewood Court
Lodi, California 95242
866-213-5836
www.neoforenxisbooks.com

ORDERING INFORMATION
Quantity sales. Special discounts are available on quantity purchases by corporations, associations, and others. For details, contact the "Special Sales Department" at the address above.

Orders by U.S. trade bookstores and wholesalers. Please contact Cardinal Publishers Group: Tel: (800) 296-0481; Fax: (317) 879-0872; Web: http://www.cardinalpub.com.

Printed in the United States of America

Publisher's Cataloging-in-Publication data
Omalu, Bennet I.
    Play hard, die young : football dementia, depression, and death /
    Bennet Omalu, M.D.
    p. cm.
    Includes bibliographical references and index.
    ISBN 978-0-9800395-0-4
1. Football injuries. 2. Head injuries. 3. Athletic injuries. 4. Brain
    concussion. 5. Sports injuries. 6. Brain—Concussion—
    Complications.
RC1220.F6 O48 2008
617.102722—dc22   2007938949

Cover and text design by Mayapriya Long, Bookwrights

FIRST EDITION
11 10 09 08   10 9 8 7 6 5 4 3 2

To Chris Nowinski,
for his courage in drawing national
attention to concussions in football.

To Mike Webster, Terry Long, and Andre Waters:
In life you offered us so much joy with your play.
In death you offered us so much more; you offered us
knowledge and taught us what we had long overlooked.

Thank you so much.

Rest in peace.

INTRODUCTION

HOW AND WHY I BECAME INVOLVED WITH THE BRAINS OF FOOTBALL PLAYERS

L ittle did I know growing up in a small town in Nigeria that I was going to end up as a forensic pathologist, but here I am. After my residency and fellowship training in four fields of pathology in July 2002, I began performing over 400 autopsies and examining over 130 brains annually.

Sometime in September 2002, I was doing my routine work, performing an autopsy on a retired National Football League player, Mike Webster. He had manifested a clinical history that resembled dementia after his retirement from the NFL. His brain appeared normal. But my combined knowledge of forensic pathology and neuropathology told me differently. Fortunately, I was trained to recognize that when an individual's brain has been damaged by repeated concussions or punches, it may still appear normal to the naked eye. I saved Mike Webster's brain in formalin and examined it comprehensively with a broad variety of tissue antibodies approximately two weeks later. My fears were confirmed. Mike suffered from a form of dementia, induced from repeated concussions sustained by playing football. He was fifty years old.

Barely three years later, in June 2005, I was back at my routine and somewhat boring post when another retired NFL player died. He had committed suicide. Lo and behold, his normal-appearing brain was at my workstation. Tissue antibody analyses confirmed that he had a type of dementia caused by repeated concussions sustained from playing football. Barely one year later, the brain remnants of a third NFL player were on my bench; for the third time, tissue analyses confirmed a type of dementia caused by repeated concussions sustained from playing football.

I've been asked why I'm the only forensic pathologist who has examined the brains of retired NFL players and identified this specific type of football-induced dementia. My answer is twofold. First, my medical background and training placed me at the right place at the right time and equipped me to recognize these cases and these diseases when I saw them. What the mind does not know, the eyes do not see. Second, as a devout Catholic, I believe in divine intervention and provenance, and I believe that the will of God always prevails. I strongly believe that God in his infinite wisdom ordained events to unfold the way they did in the fullness of time. Everything good or bad that happens in our lives happens for a reason, which may not necessarily be obvious to our mortal minds. Only God knows and understands the reasons, and if we were to know, we would become gods ourselves. Fortunately, we are not gods.

No matter the reasons, I relied on my background and training for the courage to step forward, report these cases, and publish them in a reputable medical journal. As expected, they generated widespread national and international interest and subsequent discourse on the delayed and deleterious effects of repeated concussions in football. We suddenly realized the obvious: if you want to maintain your intelligence quotient (IQ) or improve your exam scores, you do not go banging your helmeted head repeatedly on any surface, be it the turf or another player's head. At last the NFL was woken up from its deep slumber regarding the dangers of delayed, chronic brain damage caused by the game of football, dangers that had long been either denied or neglected, by fault or default.

Growing up in Africa, I did not know a lot about American football. Soccer was the most popular game in Nigeria because of its simplicity and affordability. Poor kids do not need money to enjoy a game of soccer; all that's required are bare feet, an object to kick around, and some open space. The average kid from a middle-class family in the Africa I grew up in could not afford the relatively expensive gear required to play American football. As a child I was aware of the existence of American football because I watched a few games on satellite television and saw pictures of players and games in *Time* magazine and *Ebony* magazine.

I understood it to be a game without a goal, with the players gathered up like extraterrestrials running around a large field and tackling one another, sometimes in a ferocious manner. I played organized soccer in boarding school, and I was a goalkeeper. At the same time I participated in track events like the 100-meter dash, the 4x100-meter relay, and the 200 meters. I was one of the fastest students in my boarding school, sprinting 100 meters in 10.3 seconds when I was only fourteen years old.

When I performed my first autopsy on a retired NFL player, I had been in the United States for eight years, yet I had not learned a lot about football. By this time I had a better appreciation of the game; at least I knew about the quarterback being the key player on a team. However, I had not realized that football was to America what soccer was to England or to Brazil, if not more so. American football was synonymous with the American way of life. I may have been more objective in approaching and treating the NFL cases I prosecuted because of my lack of sentimental involvement with football. Maybe if I had grown up in the United States I would have been more sentimentally inclined to these cases, and would probably have turned the other way without examining their brains, knowing that my findings might have a remote chance to undermine the game that means a lot to America. Who knows? After all is said and done, my efforts are not about me; they are about the safety of players, the families and loved ones of these players, and the scientific truth.

PART ONE

MY
PROFESSIONAL
OPINION

1

IT TOOK US BY
SURPRISE!

Modern American football originated from rugby in the second half of the nineteenth century. Rugby itself evolved from soccer. The metamorphosis of football from rugby and soccer was principally steered by students and faculty of Ivy League universities who played the early games and wrote the original rules. Formal, collective rules for American football were first written in 1876, and the American Professional Football Conference was formed in Canton, Ohio, on August 20, 1920. This name was later changed to the National Football League (NFL) on June 24, 1922. At this time the league fielded eighteen teams.

Players and coaches in the early days of American football recognized the dangerous effects of concussions sustained from playing the game. Glenn "Pop" Warner (1871–1954), a member of the College Football Hall of Fame, was one of the most successful coaches in college football history, having served as a head coach for forty-four years. As far back as 1912, when some players were facing the introduction of helmets to football, good old "Pop" counseled his college football players in Carlisle, Pennsylvania, that "playing without helmets gives players more confidence, saves their head from many hard jolts and keeps their ears from becoming torn or sore. I do not encourage their use. I have never seen an accident to the head which was serious, but I have many times seen cases when hard bumps on the head so dazed the player receiving them that he lost his memory for a time and had to be removed from the game."

Admiral Joseph Mason "Bull" Reeves (1872–1948) was the father of carrier aviation in the U.S. Navy. He integrated aircraft carriers into the U.S. naval fleet, giving the navy more attack capacity. In his younger days at the Naval Academy, which he joined in 1890, Admiral Reeves became a heroic football player; in those days American football players did not wear helmets. He suffered so many blows to his head that a navy doctor warned him that he would risk death or instant insanity if he received another kick to his head. Admiral Reeves asked a shoemaker to create a leather helmet for him, which he wore for an Army-Navy game in 1893. Reeves' equipment is considered to be the first football helmet, and he is often credited with its invention.

As football passed through its early developmental phases and maturation, the helmet was deemed the saving contraption that would protect football players from all types of head and brain injuries, including abrasions, contusions, and lacerations of the scalp; fractures of the skull; intracranial hemorrhages, and contusions and lacerations of the brain. Although many players thought wearing helmets was not a manly thing to do, the professional league encouraged their use. By 1940, when the NFL made wearing helmets mandatory, a great majority of the professional players had long since taken to wearing them anyway. The year 1940 is cited as the last time a professional NFL player played in a game without wearing a helmet.

The designs and material compositions of the helmet passed through many biomechanical and materials-science modifications, adaptations, and state-of-the-art innovations as science and technology advanced into the twenty-first century. The helmet by the 1970s had become a highly sophisticated and technologically advanced piece of equipment that did a marvelous job of protecting players from severe and direct injuries to the head, skull, and brain. The occurrence of these types of injuries in the NFL was reduced to a minimum. Life-threatening fractures of the skull or bleeding inside the skull and brain became almost nonexistent. The NFL deserves credit for doing an excellent job in this regard, especially for instituting additional rule changes that further reduced the incidence of head injuries. By 1974 helmets were becoming thicker, more sophisticated, and more rigid. Suffice it to say, though, that the sense of security was false indeed.

Back in Pop Warner's day, players would be removed from play because of diminished sensorium and loss of memory following hard bumps to the head. Becoming dazed in a game of football was not a big deal. Complaining about concussions of the brain was not expected, and if you could not play through concussions, then you were not tough enough to remain a football player. This culture carried over to the early NFL. Players

were either uninformed or ill-informed about the dangers
of concussions and subconcussions. Since most concussions were not dramatic, life-ending injuries and were not
sufficient attention-grabbers, the play of the game, the flow
of adrenalin, and the flow of money all continued. Players
who suffered severe concussions were taken out of play for
a short while and then returned back to play as soon as
possible. The wisdom at that time was that resting a player who may have suffered a severe concussion for several
days to several weeks would be curative and that the injury
would not result in significant, permanent brain damage.
That thinking was as wrong as it could be. The pageantry of
football matches the spectacle of the ancient Roman gladi-
atorial events and is attended by myriad injuries, the most
frequent of which involve the brain and have the capacity to
cause permanent brain damage.

Not until the 1990s, after repeated concussions and
their deleterious outcomes compelled many players to retire, did the NFL realize that there were many more questions than answers. In 1994 the NFL commissioned a Mild
Traumatic Brain Injury (MTBI) committee to address the
issue of concussions. Unfortunately, while yielding many
scientific papers on the biomechanics and immediate outcomes of football brain injuries, the committee's laudable
efforts ignored the possible long-term and delayed effects
of repeated concussions or subconcussions. In fact, some
of the scientific papers of the MTBI committee claimed that
repeated concussions and prompt return to play after concussions had no long-term damaging effects to the brain.
Again they were as wrong as they could have been.

The mandatory use of helmets by football players and

the changes of some rules of the game had addressed and progressively mitigated the incidence of some types of fatal and severe head injuries sustained during the play of football. While we congratulated ourselves on the biotechnological successes of modern helmet design, a long-defined but subtle disease reemerged like a thief in the night. While we slumbered, this disease stole some of our beloved professional football players away. There was a sudden national reawakening. Some of us were in denial, some were surprised or pretended to be surprised, and some were simply astonished.

Boxing—like football, a pursuit of intense and violent contact—is a very old sport, traceable to ancient times. Boxing became an Olympic sport in ancient Greece in 688 BC and thrived on a large scale during the reign of the Roman Empire, but its prominence fell with that of Rome. Modern boxing was revived in England in the early 1700s and became a professional sport. Dr. Harrison Stanley Martland, a forensic pathologist from Newark, New Jersey, and the first chief medical examiner of Essex County, New Jersey, described in 1928 a disease in boxers that he called punch-drunk syndrome, later called dementia pugilistica. Symptoms resembled a combination of Parkinson's disease and Alzheimer's disease and occurred in young boxers who were in their twenties and thirties. While the boxers who suffer from dementia pugilistica are "drunk" from repeated punches, football players who suffer from gridiron dementia are "drunk" from repeated concussions. This dementia, which is presenting in former football players in their forties and fifties, resembles tangle-only dementia, which typically occurs in people in their eighties and nineties.

Dr. Martland's epochal paper created tremendous controversy in medicine, sports, government, and politics. Professional boxers were elusive about their experiences, and autopsies of boxers were extremely rare. The few published studies of dementia pugilistica comprised case reports, case series, and groupings of reports based on the investigation of the brains of a few ex-boxers. Following mounting public interest and debates, the House of Lords of England, in 1962, referred the question of the medical aspects of boxing to the Royal College of Physicians of London (ironically, this bill was sponsored by a member of the house named Lord Brain). Not until 1969 did a report by the Royal College confirm the danger of chronic brain damage occurring in boxers as a result of their careers. Since 1969, thousands of scientific papers and research studies have confirmed that all types of contact sports can result in chronic brain damage, dementia, cognitive impairment, loss of memory, and major depression.

For some reason, people who played and organized American football were not listening, refused to listen, were in denial, or simply turned the other way, probably because of what football means to the United States. Football is big money, big fun, and the soul of America. No one who truly loves football would want to recognize anything negative about the sport. But no matter how we try to deny it, the truth will always prevail. Ironically, the same scenario that was played out in the boxing sociopolitical arena of the twentieth century is being replayed in the context of football in the twenty-first century. The first case of dementia in a football player generated controversy. The most outspoken critics and skeptics were physicians associated with the NFL, hired and paid by the league. They denied the existence of this disease and claimed that the observation of gridiron dementia was probably a misrepresentation, a random anomaly, or an aberration. As with boxers, professional football players are elusive about their experiences, and autopsies of football players are extremely rare. At the beginning we would expect to find only one or two case reports and case series of the autopsy evidence of this disease. Yet preliminary, large-scale, questionnaire-based studies have confirmed that football players as a cohort of the general population may be at least three to five times more likely to develop dementia and major depression than the general population. In 2007, we obviously do not need the U.S. Congress to become an arbiter, as the House of Lords became in boxing, to confirm the danger of chronic brain damage occurring in football players as a result of their careers.

Gridiron dementia does not occur in every professional football player, just as dementia pugilistica occurs in perhaps only about 20 percent of retired professional boxers. The boxers who suffer dementia pugilistica may exhibit progressive deterioration and a slowing and loss of brain functioning, including loss of memory, loss of language, and loss of executive functioning—needed for activities such as business and money management. They also may develop accompanying psychiatric disorders such as major depression, suicidal ideation, suicide, paranoia, confusional states, explosive behaviors, and social phobias. Why some athletes would develop these diseases and others would not should eventually be elucidated by science, but the existence of these diseases cannot be denied.

By serendipity, I examined two and one-tenth brains of three retired NFL players between 2002 and 2006. These brains revealed some tissue findings that were similar to the tissue findings of dementia pugilistica. After retirement from the NFL, these three players suffered from bizarre behaviors, major depression, progressive deterioration of brain functioning, and progressive deterioration in socio-economic status. All three players had made multiple suicide attempts, and two eventually succeeded. They all died broke and in debt, having lost multimillions of dollars in savings and assets. The recurrent questions were: Can a disease similar to dementia pugilistica occur in football players? If yes, why was it not discovered earlier and why now? Could there have been a cover-up or a screw-up? Looking back in time we begin to wonder why many retired NFL players decline from the prominence of professional play to oblivion, and sometimes destitution, in retirement.

Amateur and professional athletes sustain brain injuries from three categories of sports:

1. Contact sports like boxing and martial arts, in which impact to the head is integral to the play
2. Contact sports like football, rugby, hockey, and lacrosse, in which impact to the head is incidental to

the play

3. Lower-contact sports like soccer, baseball, and bas-
   ketball, in which impact to the head is accidental to
   the play

Dementia, neuropsychological deficits, and psychiatric disorders are well-established sequelae of all types of
brain injuries sustained from contact sports. One would expect that given the confirmed association between contact
sports, brain injury, and delayed sequelae of brain injury, a
program should have been in place whereby all retired NFL
players were monitored and followed up for the development of dementia and major depression, especially when
there were remotely established concussion precedents in
the history of football in the United States. However, by the
end of 2006 no such program existed. What existed were
episodic news and stories of one retired NFL player or the
other who had been forced to retire because of brain injury;
who had lost all his money or his business following retirement; who had been admitted to a nursing home for dementia patients; who had suffered from memory loss, cognitive
impairment, and major depression; or who was suffering
from constant headaches.

In death, the brains of three retired NFL players revealed
the underlying truth to us more than eighty years after the
American Professional Football Conference was formed in
1920. These brains reminded us that football players can
suffer from trauma-induced organic brain disease and can
develop gridiron dementia, a disease that resembles but is
distinct from dementia pugilistica. Is gridiron dementia re-

sponsible for the abnormal and bizarre behaviors we have observed in many retired NFL players? Is gridiron dementia responsible for many retired NFL players doing poorly in business, losing all their hard-earned millions of dollars, and even becoming destitute? Is gridiron dementia responsible for many retired NFL players suffering from major depression, breaking up intimate social relationships, and even committing suicide? If so, who are the NFL players who will develop gridiron dementia and why? Will high-school, college, and amateur football players develop the same disease?

2

WHY WOULD A FOOTBALL PLAYER SUFFER FROM DEMENTIA AND MAJOR DEPRESSION?

American football is an extremely exciting, adrenaline-charged, and brutal game. Likewise, football players are extremely tough and strong people. They are tough and strong in the body, mind, and spirit, and they must remain tough and strong to keep playing football. The game of football entails high levels of kinetic energy, movement, contact, and impact between players. Large amounts of kinetic energy are transferred to the bodies of players while they play. This transference of kinetic energy to the body is called biomechanical loading, of which there are two types: impact biomechanical loading and impulsive biomechanical loading

In impact biomechanical loading, kinetic energy is transferred to the body of a player from direct impact with an unyielding hard or firm surface, like another player or the ground. Contact defines this form of biomechanical loading. In impulsive biomechanical loading, kinetic energy is transferred to the body without direct contact with any surface, such as by sudden changes in motion via acceleration or deceleration.

The body part most vulnerable to biomechanical loading is the head because it is connected to the rest of the body by a highly mobile neck. The organ in the body that is most vulnerable to biomechanical loading is the brain, due to the unique anatomy of the skull and the brain. The consistency of the normal brain is semisolid and may be akin to a colloidal gel, Jell-O, or thick custard. The brain practically floats inside the cavity of the skull and can move and oscillate freely, often impacting the inner surfaces of the skull bones during all forms of biomechanical loading.

Impact and impulsive biomechanical loading are not mutually exclusive. They can occur together and can accentuate each other in a game of football. Imagine that player X is running fast with the ball and is tackled by player Y. Player Y's helmet impacts player X's helmet, causing impact biomechanical loading of both players' heads. The tackle and impact by player Y makes player X, who was running fast, stop suddenly and fall to the ground, causing a sudden change in motion from high acceleration to sudden deceleration within a matter of seconds. The acceleration-deceleration effect causes a secondary impulsive biomechanical loading of both players' brains, especially player X's, since he was running at a higher velocity and acceleration.

One of the outcomes of biomechanical loading is shearing of the brain, which is the underlying mechanism of the concussion injury. The brain is very vulnerable to shearing forces because of the biological makeup of brain tissue. Water constitutes 75 to 80 percent of the human brain. The unique microscopic anatomy of the brain makes it extremely vulnerable to levels of shearing that would not affect other organs in the body. The brain contains approximately 100 billion nerve cells distributed over more than one hundred distinct groups called nuclei. Other types of cells that support nerve cells number over 300 billion. Each nerve cell measures five to one hundred micron-meters in diameter, and each brain cell sends out microscopic nerve fibers to more than one other brain cell. A nerve fiber can measure from micron-meters to millimeters and even up to one meter in length, and from nanometers to micron-meters in thickness. There are therefore hundreds of billions if not trillions of nerve fibers and nerve cells in the brain literally floating freely in water. For individual structural support and stability, therefore, nerve fibers contain membranes and microskeletons, which are made up of certain types of proteins (for example, amyloid protein and tau protein).

The human head and neck have a greater anatomic capacity for nodding movements forward and backward in a linear fashion than for movements sideways in a rotational or angular fashion. Therefore, any biomechanical loading that induces angular or rotational acceleration-deceleration of the head is more deleterious and lethal than biomechanical loading that induces linear acceleration-deceleration of the head. Unfortunately a great majority of biomechanical loadings suffered by football players induce angular-rotational acceleration-deceleration of the brain.

A football player can sustain impacts at a velocity of 25 miles per hour, and rapid changes in head and brain velocity can reach 20.1 miles per hour during a game of football. Peak head and brain acceleration-deceleration during a concussion can reach 138 gravitational (g) force and can last for up to fifteen milliseconds. One g force is equal to the force of gravity. Thus, a football player's brain can sustain forces from a concussion that are up to 138 times the force of gravity. These are extremely high levels of force for a brain that is made up of 75 to 80 percent water. In most cases, impact to a helmeted head during a game of football does not generate any external injuries to the head like scratches, bruises, or cuts. Kinetic energy is not dissipated on the surface of the head to cause external injury. The energy is dumped on the brain inside the skull.

Diffuse shearing of the brain by high levels of energy manifests clinically in a variety of symptoms, that are characteristic of concussions. A concussion is clinically defined as a clinical syndrome resulting from mechanical force, which is characterized by immediate or transient alteration in brain function, including alteration of mental status and level of consciousness. Immediately following a concussion, a football player may manifest alteration of awareness or consciousness and even loss of consciousness, a ding, sensations of being dazed or stunned, sensations of wooziness or fogginess, a seizure, or loss of memory. Hours to days and weeks after a concussion, a player may still manifest persistent headaches, dizziness, lightheadedness, drowsiness, loss of balance, unsteadiness, fainting attacks, cognitive dysfunction, memory loss, hearing loss, ringing noise in the ear, blurred vision, double vision, visual loss, personality changes, lethargy, fatigue, and inability to perform usual daily activities.

There is no such thing as a minor concussion, although some concussions are more acutely devastating than others. No single concussion of the brain should be taken lightly, especially when there are approximately three hundred thousand concussions suffered by professional football players per season in the United States. There are 1.6 to 3.8 million sports-related and recreation-related concussions and traumatic brain injuries suffered in the United States annually, with the vast majority going unreported, undocumented, and untreated. Each NFL team incurs at least one concussion per game of football and possibly incurs additional concussions from practice. A repeat concussion following an earlier concussion within minutes, hours, days, or even weeks does not have to be severe for its effects to be deadly or permanently disabling. This phenomenon is called second impact syndrome, and this is why football players are sometimes taken out of play by a team's physician or coach for a period that is determined by the physician or coach. But the pertinent question is: how long after suffering a concussion should a player wait to return to play?

Concussion of the brain physically disrupts and shears the delicately balanced milieu of the brain cells and nerve fibers. The microskeleton of the brain cells and nerve fibers are physically disrupted by each and every concussion. Concussions involving extreme levels of force can literally tear so many nerve fibers (diffuse axonal injury) that immediate death or permanent brain damage results. Concussions involving lower levels of force can disrupt the microskeleton of the brain cells and nerve fibers without tearing the cells and nerves. In this instance, the effects, signs, and symptoms of the concussion are transient, remaining until the brain cells sufficiently repair and heal themselves. The effects of a repeat concussion before the brain cells are sufficiently healed will be accentuated and will cause exponentially greater damage. For this reason, a relatively mild and innocuous repeat concussion after a previous concussion (second impact syndrome) can precipitate immediate death.

The treatment for concussion is rest and withdrawal from play to avoid a repeat concussion. The principle behind the rest is to allow the brain cells and nerves sufficient time to repair and heal themselves. Sometimes nonsteroidal analgesics are given to the players to relieve headaches and pain. Football players who sustain concussions are clinically assessed immediately to determine the severity, but there is no universal agreement on the grades of severity. Consequently, different guidelines have arisen for the evaluation of concussions and return-to-play decisions for professional athletes. However, most clinical guidelines recognize three different grades of concussions and share similar recommendations for return to play. The two sets of guidelines that are most followed in the United States were formulated by the American Academy of Neurology (AAN) and by Dr. Robert C. Cantu, one of the world's most prominent and accomplished sports physicians and neurosurgeons.

In 1986, Dr. Cantu formulated a set of guidelines that was later adopted by the American College of Sports Medicine. The Cantu guidelines are the most commonly used and well-known guidelines for concussion diagnosis and management. According to the Cantu guidelines, *grade I (mild) concussions* are not associated with loss of consciousness; posttraumatic amnesia is absent or is less than thirty minutes in duration, or postconcussion signs and symptoms last less than thirty minutes. Football players who suffer their first grade I concussion may return to play when asymptomatic for one week. For the second grade I concussion, they return to play in two weeks if asymptomatic for one week. For the third grade I concussion, they are terminated for the next season and may return to play the next season if asymptomatic.

Grade II (moderate) concussions are associated with loss of consciousness lasting less than one minute, posttraumatic amnesia lasting longer than thirty minutes but less than twenty-four hours, or postconcussion signs and symptoms lasting longer than thirty minutes but less than twenty-four hours. Football players who suffer their first grade II concussion may return to play one week after being asymptomatic. For the second grade II concussion, they stay out of play for a minimum of one month and may return to play then if asymptomatic for one week. They may be considered for the termination of the season. For the third grade II concussion, they are terminated for the season and may return to play the following season if asymptomatic.

Grade III (severe) concussions are associated with loss of consciousness lasting longer than one minute or posttraumatic amnesia lasting longer than twenty-four hours or postconcussion signs and symptoms lasting longer than one week. Football players who suffer their first grade III concussion may return to play after a minimum of one month after the injury and may then return to play if asymptomatic for one week. For the second grade III concussion, they are terminated for the season and may return to play the next season if asymptomatic. They may be discouraged from returning to football.

In all three grades of concussions, asymptomatic means without postconcussion symptoms, including loss of memory (amnesia), at rest or with exertion. As it seems, football players with repeated concussions are recommended to be sidelined for longer periods of time and possibly not allowed to play for the remainder of the season or discouraged from continuing to play football.

The death of several Colorado high school football players prompted the Colorado Medical Society to formulate, in 1991, more restrictive guidelines for the assessment and treatment of concussions. The Colorado guidelines were later adopted by the National Collegiate Athletic Association (NCAA). More recently other sets of guidelines have been proposed, but no consensus within the sports medicine community exists as to which set of guidelines is the most appropriate.

The brains of boxers who suffer from dementia pugilistica, the brains of three retired NFL players, and the lives of other retired football players who have suffered from dementia are telling us that the way we look at concussions may not be correct. These brains and lives are telling us that certain types of individuals may not recover completely from concussions. Obvious clinical signs and symptoms may not be grossly present, but the brain cells may not recover biochemically at the subcellular level. There may be a threshold for the number or severity of concussions each football player's brain cells may tolerate, and once this threshold is surpassed, the brain cells may not have the innate capacity to completely repair and heal themselves following shearing of their microskeleton.

Brain cells may not have unlimited reserve or capacity to heal themselves following multiple and repeated concussions. A concussion causes physical damage to brain cells and places demands on the biochemical repair mechanisms of brain cells. Repeated concussions are more likely to cause additive and cumulative damages to the brain cells, and at some threshold the brain cells will progressively lose the ability to completely heal themselves. This progressive loss of biochemical repair capacity results in the loss of the brain cells' ability to process membrane and microskeletal proteins (like amyloid protein and tau protein). Abnormal forms of these proteins begin to accumulate in the brain and begin to take up abnormal conformations in the brain cells (amyloid plaques, neurofibrillary tangles, and neuritic threads). These abnormal proteins are toxic to the brain cells and eventually begin to kill off the brain cells in a

progressive, unrelenting manner. The accumulation of abnormal proteins and the loss of brain cells are responsible
for the development of dementia, neuropsychiatric impairment, and major depression in football players. All these
diseases are combined into one syndrome called chronic
traumatic encephalopathy (CTE). The type of CTE found in
boxers is called dementia pugilistica or punch-drunk syndrome. The type of CTE found in football players is called
gridiron dementia or concussion-drunk syndrome. A young
retired football player who has gridiron dementia in his
thirties, forties, or fifties will have a brain resembling the
brain of a dementia-afflicted individual who is over eighty
years old.

The disease model of gridiron dementia resembles
the disease model of mesothelioma (cancer of the lining
of the lungs) due to occupational exposure to asbestos.
Mesothelioma occurs in retired asbestos workers after a very
long latent period, which can range from ten to seventy-
five years. The risk of developing mesothelioma correlates
with the age and time of first exposure to asbestos and
with the duration and cumulative exposure to asbestos.
Following cessation of exposure to asbestos deleterious
biochemical and molecular responses to the asbestos fibers
continue and progress to the development of a cancer many
years later. Gridiron dementia possesses a similar disease
model. The deleterious effects of repeated concussions to
the brain cells and nerve fibers are additive and cumulative. The risk of developing gridiron dementia should cor-
relate with the age at first concussion, with the cumulative
number of concussions, and with the duration of lifetime

play of football. Following cessation of play, deleterious biochemical and molecular responses of brain cells continue, and after a long latent period, a football player may develop gridiron dementia.

No single concussion is safe regarding the risk of developing gridiron dementia. Dementias that resemble Alzheimer's disease can develop in anyone's brain following one single episode of severe traumatic brain injury. This fact applies to everyone who suffers even one episode of severe traumatic brain injury, including football players. Changes similar to Alzheimer's disease can occur in everyone's brain, including the brain of a football player, following repeated episodes of mild traumatic brain injury like concussions. The key questions are: who is at risk of developing gridiron dementia, and what are the characteristics of players who will eventually develop gridiron dementia? We currently do not know the answers to these questions. The major shift in scientific thought is that seemingly innocuous blows to the head during the play of football, which may not be recognized by the players themselves or the team physicians, may not be innocuous after all, especially in the long term.

Over several or many years of playing football, repeated unnoticed impacts to the head and seemingly uneventful blows to the head, which are part of the game, may in the long term unknowingly induce permanent damage to the biochemical functioning of the brain cells and result in gridiron dementia. Unfortunately, this may happen after a long latent period, when the high school, college, or professional football player has moved on in life and football has become only a memory.

Given the disease model of gridiron dementia, the practice of assessing players and grouping them into Cantu's three grades of concussions in view of determining their return-to-play status may be flawed. Based upon Cantu's guidelines and other concussion guidelines, the assumption that a football player's brain recovers completely after a short rest following every concussion may not be completely true, at least in certain football players. The brains of three NFL players, the brains of boxers with dementia pugilistica, and the lives of retired NFL players who have suffered from dementia may challenge the premise of these return-to-play assumptions and concepts. Although a football player may be asymptomatic after sustaining a concussion, it may not mean that his brain cells have completely recovered from the deleterious biochemical and cellular effects of concussions even after one episode of a grade I concussion. The deleterious biochemical effects of concussions may continue on the subcellular level and may manifest as one form of brain dysfunction or the other many years later.

Experts agree on the accentuating, multiplicative, deleterious, and possibly lethal effects of a second minimal concussion shortly following a first concussion (second impact syndrome). There is therefore no reason to deny the cumulative, accentuating, multiplicative, and deleterious effects of third, fourth, fifth, sixth, and more repeated concussions over time. There is no reason that we should not have third impact syndrome, fourth impact syndrome, fifth impact syndrome, and repeated multiple impact syndrome. The repeated, multiple impact syndrome will eventually manifest as gridiron dementia or concussion-drunk syndrome.

Rather than debating the existence or nonexistence of gridiron dementia, we should focus on its human risk management. The critical issue in the risk management of gridiron dementia is the identification of football players whose brain cells are less likely to recover completely following concussions. Perhaps every player's brain cells do not completely recover biochemically following concussions. We do not really know. However, when we can identify players who may possess higher innate risk levels for gridiron dementia, such players may be advised not to play football. Such players may be taken out of play completely after just one concussion if they elect to play football. Even if we concentrate on the reported and clinically visible concussions, what about those seemingly innocuous, unnoticed blows to the head that are integral to the play of football and cause repeated subconcussions? Could these repeated subconcussions eventually contribute to the underlying causal cascades of gridiron dementia? Possibly, and why not?

3

WHAT TWO AND ONE-TENTH BRAINS TAUGHT US ABOUT DEMENTIA AND SUICIDE

Serendipity. What a big word! I encountered this word in my second year of medical school. I was not very interested in understanding what the word meant until eight years later when I was completing my residency. I began to encounter the word more often in my readings, which were progressively becoming too sophisticated for my, in many ways, uneducated brain. I finally checked it out in *Merriam-Webster's Collegiate Dictionary*, which described "serendipity" as "the faculty or phenomenon of finding valuable or agreeable things not sought for." I interpreted this to mean accidental discovery. Ironically, many years later,

I was serendipitously situated, because of my educational background and pursuits, to identify gridiron dementia in the brains of three retired NFL players who had died relatively young.

Two whole brains were examined from the first two cases. Pieces of brain tissue, which represented approximately one-tenth of the whole brain, were examined from the third case. These two and one-tenth brains revealed the same abnormalities that are typically found in the brains of elderly patients with certain types of dementias. One such dementia is tangle-only dementia, which occurs in people in their eighties and nineties. Amazingly, these three NFL players were aged only fifty, forty-five, and forty-four years old, respectively. The three players all played college football (and two also played football in high school). They were drafted into the NFL at the respective ages of twenty-two, twenty-five, and twenty-two, and they played in the NFL for seventeen, eight, and twelve years, respectively. They died approximately twelve years, twelve years, and eleven years, respectively, after retirement from the NFL.

Two major distinct abnormalities were found in these three brains. The first abnormality was the accumulation of abnormal proteins in the brain (amyloid and tau proteins), which created abnormal conformations (amyloid plaques, neurofibrillary tangles, and neuritic threads). The second distinct abnormality was significant loss and death of brain cells over all the regions of the brain. These abnormalities explained the abnormal behaviors these players each exhibited in the years before they died. Similar changes are found in the brains of retired boxers who suffer from dementia pugilistica.

Following retirement from the NFL, all three players lost all their hard-earned savings of millions of dollars. They performed very poorly in business and eventually failed in all their business endeavors. They all suffered from major depression. They all attempted suicide. Two eventually succeeded in committing suicide. One consumed ethylene glycol (antifreeze); the other shot himself in the mouth. They all died broke and in debt. In fact, one of the players was destitute at some points in his life after retirement from the NFL. He lived in a train station at one point and in his pickup truck at another.

There is unquestionable medical evidence that these three NFL players suffered from cognitive impairment and dementia. Major depression is associated with dementia. Major depression is also associated with traumatic brain injury and concussions in retired contact-sport athletes, including football players. Loss of executive functioning also accompanies major depression in football players who suffer from dementia due to repeated concussions. Loss of executive functioning refers to a progressive loss of the ability to embark on complex cognitive and intellectual tasks, like managing a business or investing and managing money. The brain cells are dying, and the residual brain cells are not performing optimally due to the presence of accumulated abnormal proteins in the brain. The final outcome is a demented, depressed man who is broke and may commit suicide. Certain parts of the brain control our emotions and mood, and certain parts of the brain secrete chemicals that maintain our emotions and mood. The brains of these three retired NFL players revealed loss of brain cells and accumulations of abnormal proteins and forms of proteins in these regions of the brain. These tissue findings explain the underlying causes of major depression and other possible neuropsychiatric symptoms that ex-NFL players with gridiron dementia may manifest.

Unfortunately, there currently exits no definitive curative drug therapy for the dementia and major depression that occur in football players. Hopefully (by serendipity or focused research) we will discover a drug that will cure dementias and major depression in retired football players and other contact-sport players. Empirical research on rats and mice may have shown already that some types of drugs could prevent or impede the formation of abnormal proteins in these animals when they are subjected to repeated concussions. These findings are still in the preliminary research stages and have not been confirmed in humans.

Another pertinent lesson that these two and one-tenth brains have taught us is that players suffering from gridiron dementia may have brains that appear grossly normal when studied with the naked eye. That is, CT scans or MRI studies of the brains of players suffering from gridiron dementia may appear unremarkable. Radiologic examinations of a retired NFL player, which indicate a normal-appearing brain, thus should not exclude a diagnosis of gridiron dementia. Direct tissue analysis of the brain still remains the gold standard for the definitive diagnosis of dementias, including gridiron dementia.

There are sociopolitical and medico-legal ramifications in regard to determining the cause and manner of death of retired football players who commit suicide and whose autopsies confirm the presence of gridiron dementia. Cause of death may be defined as the underlying factor, event, or disease that initiates or instigates a terminal chain of events that finally culminates in death, no matter the time interval between the underlying instigator of fatal events and death itself. Events that link the underlying instigator of fatal events to death constitute the mechanisms of death. The manner of death describes the circumstances or scenarios that surround the underlying cause of death. Suicide is a manner of death whereby an individual intentionally terminates his or her life by a self-inflicted injury. The cause of a suicidal death can be any type of injury.

In the instance of a football player who manifests gridiron dementia and eventually commits suicide, the mechanism of death is a suicidal act. The underlying cause of death that instigated the terminal chain of events—that is, dementia and a suicidal act—would be repeated concussions sustained from playing football. Repeated concussions are traumatic and accidental circumstances of injury sustenance. Therefore, the death of a retired football player who commits suicide as a result of gridiron dementia should rightfully be classified as accidental and not as a suicidal manner of death. For this rule to hold, an autopsy must be performed, and the brain must be examined for the presence of pathognomonic tissue changes of gridiron dementia.

Stigma is attached to depression and suicide in most modern societies, including the American society. Depression and suicide are diseases that people neither are proud of nor want to be associated with. The social trauma inflicted on the family and loved ones of a suicide victim can be unimaginably painful. Football players who suffer from gridiron dementia and end up committing suicide may not kill themselves because of some natural mental disease but rather because of an unnatural trauma-induced disease. They may kill themselves because of the final outcomes of repeated brain concussions they sustained from playing football. These football players and their families should not be victimized any further by classifying these deaths as suicides. The suicidal acts in these instances constitute the final, terminal mechanisms of death and not the underlying causes of death. The underlying cause of death should be viewed as gridiron dementia due to repeated traumatic brain injuries. These deaths should be classified as accidental deaths since the suicidal act was instigated by traumatic brain injuries and not by a natural mental disorder.

4

THE RESPONSE
OF THE NATIONAL
FOOTBALL LEAGUE

The National Football League (NFL) is a highly responsible and proficient organization that has turned American football into one of the most exciting and profitable sports in the world. The league has matured with the game and has confronted different challenges and growing pains at various times in the sport's history. Most times they have done what they perceived to be best for the sport and for the league. As in every human endeavor, however, they may have fallen short of the best, their best may not have been good enough, and they may have simply overlooked certain things and done what was far from the best for the sport.

In 1994, Paul Tagliabue, the commissioner of the NFL, formed the Mild Traumatic Brain Injury (MTBI) committee to examine the issue of concussions in football. The committee later recommended that the NFL should sponsor independent scientific research into the causes, diagnosis, treatment, and prevention of concussions. These independent research projects may not have been as independent as we would have wanted them to be, since the one who pays the piper dictates the tune. A globally significant mistake was made when the six initial members of the MTBI committee were appointed; they included a neurologist, a neurosurgeon, a neuropsychologist, a biomechanical engineer, and an epidemiologist. There was no neuropathologist or an expert in the genesis or cascades of development of disease (pathogenesis). The focus of the MTBI committee expectedly drifted to the biomechanics and acute manifestations of sports-related brain trauma. They published many scientific papers on these subjects without paying any significant attention to the possible delayed effects of repeated concussions. Understandably, we are all human and we all make mistakes.

Following the diagnosis of gridiron dementia on the first retired NFL player in 2002, my colleagues and I were obliged to climb to the top of the mountain of science and announce the news to the scientific community. Our professional obligation and responsibility was to report the case in a reputable scientific journal since it would be the very first autopsy-confirmed case of dementia in a football player published in the medical literature. We chose to publish this first case in the journal *Neurosurgery* because the NFL published most of its brain trauma–related medical research in this journal, although the validity of some of the research findings has been questioned. The case was finally published in July 2005 after a drawn-out and tiring struggle to convince the reviewers and editors of the journal that the case was scientifically valid. But thankfully, and with our deep appreciation to the editorial board of the journal, especially Dr. Donald Marion, a prominent neurosurgeon, the case was finally published.

Several months after the publication of the first case, I received an e-mail from Dr. Marion requesting that I respond to an attached letter that the MTBI committee of the NFL had submitted to the journal. He called me later to discuss the NFL letter and gracefully advised me on what was expected from me. My initial response was that of fear and trepidation. I have sweated profusely out of fear on only several occasions in my life; this was one of them. I felt very intimidated by the fact that doctors who represented the almighty NFL had submitted a letter requesting the retraction of our published paper. After a gulp of my favorite whisky, I settled down, printed the letter, and perused it. First, I noticed that it was rather too lengthy for a letter to the editor in response to a published paper in a journal. Second, I noticed that it may have been even longer than the original paper that was its subject matter. Third, I noticed that it was rather too unfriendly and noncollegial, too confrontational and accusatory, and just too critical. I smiled, my heart beat much slower, and the profuse sweating stopped. Perhaps the whisky was taking effect.

I smiled because the letter from the MTBI committee was too defensive. It reeked of ulterior motive. I was surprised by this response and stance since I had presumed that the NFL would be happy with our scientific findings, which I had assumed would enhance their research and understanding of concussions. I was proven wrong. I shredded the printed copies of the letter and went about my chores for the day, hoping to deal with it some other time. I forwarded copies of the letter to my coauthors. Two weeks later I composed a response and sent it to my coauthors, who made changes before we finally submitted the response to *Neurosurgery*. The NFL letter, our response, and comments by other respected names in the field of concussions and sports-related injuries were all published in *Neurosurgery* in May 2006.

The letter from the NFL was written and signed by Drs. Elliot J. Pellman, Ira R. Casson, and David C. Viano, three of the most prominent NFL physicians. Dr. Pellman was actually the chairman of the MTBI committee. They essentially requested that our paper be retracted since it was scientifically invalid and flawed. The only papers that are retracted from publication are papers written by authors who lied or who have forged results and conclusions—that is, dubious and intentionally falsified scientific papers. Ours was not the least bit falsified. We simply reported what we saw. These NFL doctors probably wanted to set a precedent that if certain powerful and influential doctors do not like a published scientific paper, they may have it retracted. Certainly, they weren't the first group to try.

Drs. Pellman, Casson, and Viano attacked us, claiming that we seriously misinterpreted the neuropathological findings in the case and that we had a complete misunderstanding of the relevant medical literature. Neither

Dr. Pellman, Dr. Casson, nor Dr. Viano was a neuropathologist. I wondered how doctors who were not neuropathologists could interpret neuropathological findings better than neuropathologists, especially when these doctors did not think that it was prudent to appoint a neuropathologist to their committee, even in an advisory capacity. They extensively reviewed the neuropathological literature in their letter, arguing that our first case did not have gridiron dementia and did not meet the neuropathological criteria for such a diagnosis. I was extremely disappointed, for it seemed then that the NFL may have unfortunately adopted a stance of denial. I truly understand the embarrassment our report may have caused the members of the MTBI committee, but rather than adopting a stance of denial, they should have considered options more constructive than spurting a rather emotion-laden letter to the editor of *Neurosurgery*.

We replied with a more collegial and fraternal letter, recognized their "scholarly" letter, and suggested that the NFL should seriously consider our first case as a sentinel case that warranted further investigation by the NFL to confirm if there was a danger of professional football players developing chronic and irreversible brain damage. We reiterated that the NFL should begin examining the long-term effects of brain injury in its former players and volunteered to collaborate with the MTBI committee in developing and implementing an optimal research program that would address this important issue. At the time of publication of this book, almost five years later, the MTBI committee of the NFL has neither sent me a letter nor given me a phone call.

The editorial board of *Neurosurgery* did not agree with Drs. Pellman, Casson, and Viano. In response to their letter, Dr. Donald Marion wrote in part, "As members of the Mild Traumatic Brain Injury Committee of the NFL, and clinician-scientists that are clearly devoted to the investigation of sports-related concussion, Drs. Casson, Pellman, and Viano should welcome the contribution from Omalu et al. and consider the findings of that report highly relevant to their own research, rather than recommending retraction of the article." He continued, "Together with subsequent reports of autopsy results from the NFL players, which hopefully will include the important premorbid clinical details, we will begin to establish a reliable definition of chronic traumatic encephalopathy typical for professional football players." I would like to personally thank Dr. Marion for his most constructive and progressive scientific stance.

In another press interview, Dr. Elliot Pellman, who was still the chairman of the NFL MTBI committee, reiterated, "My problem is the conclusions are, from my end, speculative and unscientific." This was rather a noncollegial statement from Dr. Pellman. When we discovered the second case and the third case, when other football players were emboldened to step forward, and when other researchers published more papers to support our cases, Dr. Pellman stepped down as the chairman of the NFL MTBI committee in February 2007. This was barely three months after our paper on gridiron dementia in a second NFL player was published in *Neurosurgery*, and it was approximately one month after the third case of autopsy-confirmed gridiron dementia was reported in the *New York Times* on January 18, 2007.

Some of my colleagues and I have wondered if the NFL was adopting a strategy that may be similar to the denial or cover-up of the harmful effects of cigarette smoking by the tobacco industry. We honestly do not know. However, we know that the main focus of the NFL has been on the short-term effects of traumatic brain injury, and they have done a great job in preventing and managing brain injuries in the short term. However, by fault or default, they forgot all about long-term or delayed effects of repetitive and mild concussions over a prolonged period. Thankfully, and in the fullness of time, the brains of three great NFL players have woken us from our slumber to remind us that it is high time we shifted or broadened our focus.

In another press report, Dr. Pellman reported that the MTBI committee of the NFL had embarked on a program to study gridiron dementia in NFL players. This study would last two or three years and would involve about 160 active and retired NFL players. My opinion as an epidemiologist is that this is the wrong research methodology to adopt in studying dementia and major depression in football players. Gridiron dementia is a long-term, chronic degenerative disease of the brain that requires a longer period to study. What we need is a nationwide, multi-institutional, and multidisciplinary research project whereby all NFL players are followed up clinically and monitored for the rest of their lives. This should be an ongoing program that would set up a database on NFL players and their behavioral and mental trends. Then after many years—ten, twenty, or thirty years, or even across one or two generations—we would begin to recognize emerging trends and begin to understand this disease better. The enigma of dementia and major depression in football players cannot be deciphered by a two- or three-year study involving only selected players.

Effective February 1, 2007, two weeks after our third case of gridiron dementia was reported in the *New York Times*, the NFL and the players' union, as part of the collective bargaining agreement, established a new retirement plan called the "88 Plan" to provide medical benefits to retired NFL players who have dementia. The plan would reimburse or pay for certain costs related to dementia treatment not to exceed eighty-eight thousand dollars per year for nursing care or day care and fifty thousand dollars per year for home care. The plan was in honor of John Mackey, an NFL Hall of Famer who was a Baltimore Colts star of the 1971 Super Bowl. John Mackey was diagnosed with dementia in 2001 at the ripe age of fifty-nine. His medical costs for the management of dementia were rising, and his wife Sylvia could not keep up solely with his pension of twenty-five hundred dollars per month, even after she had sold their home in California and taken a job as a flight attendant with a national airline. The name of the plan and the maximum amount was in honor of John Mackey, whose uniform number was "88." His wife had initiated establishment of this plan when she approached the NFL commissioner to do more for NFL players. It is interesting to note that John Mackey often visits the same nursing home where Ralph Wenzel, his fellow teammate from the San Diego Chargers of 1972, lives and happens to be suffering from dementia. Nobody truly knows the number of retired NFL players who are suffering from dementia, but the grapevine has it that many of them are living in oblivion with dementia and major depression. By the end of the third month after the 88 Plan had taken effect, fifty-four retired players had applied for the plan; thirty-five had been approved, while nineteen were pending. This is a rather high number of dementia cases for a small cohort of the population.

To put the numbers in perspective, the estimated incidence of dementia in the U.S. population at ages sixty to sixty-nine is about sixty-six dementia cases per one hundred thousand people per year. Already we know of close to sixty retired NFL players who are registered with the NFL dementia plan. The amazing thing is that there are fewer than ten thousand living retired NFL players. This leaves us with an estimated prevalence of at least sixty dementia cases per ten thousand retired NFL players. The executive director of the NFL players' union, who was one of those who had denied any association between football and dementia, was allegedly taken aback when he saw the number of retired players applying for the 88 Plan. He said he had always thought that one or two players were having problems, but he did not actually realize the extent of the problem of dementia among retired NFL players. He'd better brace himself for more surprises, for the truth is coming to light.

Paradoxically, prominent doctors who represent the NFL still maintain their denial stance that gridiron dementia is not caused by playing football. In a statement he made to the press, Dr. Ira Casson, the cochair of the NFL's Committee on Mild Traumatic Brain Injury and a respected neurologist, said that he strongly disagreed with our findings and conclusions. He said vehemently that what we saw in the brains of three NFL players was not dementia pugilistica or punch-drunk syndrome. I simply could not understand Dr. Casson's seemingly mistaken assumption. Of course what we saw in the brains of three NFL players was neither dementia pugilistica nor punch-drunk syndrome, since these players were not boxers and received no punches. What we saw in these players was gridiron dementia and not dementia pugilistica. What we saw in these players was not punch-drunk syndrome, but concussion-drunk syndrome. I cannot remember the last time a football player was involved in a fistfight or received repeated punches to the head in a league game.

In a highly watched sports news documentary aired by HBO on May 14, 2007, on *Real Sports with Bryant Gumbel*, Dr. Casson was asked in six different ways if repeated concussions sustained while playing football can result in chronic brain damage, dementia, or major depression. Six times he said no, there was no association between football and chronic brain damage, dementia, or major depression. To say that I was shocked by Dr. Casson's statements would be an understatement. I wonder if the governing agency for the practice of neurology in the United States saw that program.

Since we reported our first case in July 2005, there have been countless stories and reports in the national and international news media, both print and electronic, on the issue of gridiron dementia. One news report that I thought was unique was a *Washington Post* story on April 25, 2007, titled "'Brain Chaser' Tackles Effects of NFL Hits." This story by

Les Carpenter was intended to tell the story about me as a person and my personal efforts and struggles regarding securing the brains of NFL players when they die. It was a beautiful write-up, and Les did a great job.

(I received so many positive and negative calls about this report. One call was from a young man who had played football in college. He wanted to know why the NFL had not approached me to work with or advise it on dementia in retired football players. I told him that I did not know. He said that I was a rather remarkable but unconventional guy, and the reason that the NFL had not approached me may be because I am unconventional. I thought his opinion on the phone was unconventional as well, so I asked him if he could explain what he meant. He said that from what he had read in the *Washington Post*, I was a Nigerian, I was black, I was young, and I was not American. I was not a mainstream, well-known, elderly, and established academic researcher with a track record or a history. I was a nobody. I asked him how all these things about me related to the stance of the NFL. He continued that I was from Nigeria, a country that is not known or respected for scientific breakthroughs. If I had been a Caucasian European researcher who was probably in his sixties, the NFL would have responded differently. I quickly told him that I did not understand what he was implying, asked him to have a good day, and hung up. Several days after that I considered over and over again what I heard on the phone. I could not really understand the young man's proposition. However, if there was any truth in his proposition, no matter how remotely true it could have been, then it is extremely sad and we may still have a long,

long way to go in the United States. I chose to believe that his comments and propositions were nothing but untamed and reckless assertions. I hope I was correct.)

In spring 2007, the NFL announced a national seminar of all the league's trainers and physicians on June 19, 2007, in Chicago, to discuss the issue of concussions. Some independent researchers in the field of concussions were invited to deliver presentations at the seminar. I was not aware of the seminar until Dr. Julian Bailes, one of the most prominent sports-medicine neurosurgeons in the world, who was speaking at the seminar, called to ask me if I was invited to speak at the seminar. Of course not, I told him. I was not even aware of the seminar. I had to send him all my data on the cases I had examined for him to add to his presentation and present at the seminar. I was willing to give up every bit of data I had in my possession as long as the data could be used to spread the word about the dangers of repeated concussions. What I was doing should not be about me but about the truth, the lives, and the safety of everyone who plays football. Dr. Bailes has been one of the very few doctors who have reached out to me and supported me in a very strong way to continue the good work I was doing. I admire him greatly for his courage and integrity.

On May 22, 2007, the communications and public relations offices of the NFL in New York issued a press release titled "NFL Outlines Standards for Concussion Management." Chris Nowinski e-mailed me a copy of the press release. When I reviewed the press release, the first question that went through my mind was, why is the NFL releasing this now? Is the NFL announcing standards for concussion management in 2007, eighty-seven years after the American Professional Football Conference was formed? Does it mean that all this while the NFL and its teams did not have any standards for the management of concussions? If so, why has it just decided to develop such standards despite insisting that football does not cause any significant chronic brain damage? In addition, the press release announced an updated membership of the Mild Traumatic Brain Injury Committee of the NFL with non-NFL and NFL medical doctors and doctors of philosophy. A new Retired Player Study Investigators committee was also announced. Another key question was why a study for retired football players was not initiated in 1994 when the MTBI committee of the NFL was first convened. Why did we have to wait so long until the deaths and autopsies of three retired football players prompted us to think about dementia in football players, despite systematic denials by a few that football does not cause chronic brain damage?

The 2007 MTBI committee comprised fourteen members: eight non-NFL and six NFL members. There were nine doctors, three PhDs, and two head athletic trainers from two NFL teams. The medical doctors were two neurologists, two neurosurgeons, one neuroradiologist, three sports medicine physicians, and one emergency medicine physician, and one PhD each in epidemiology, neuropsychology, and biomedical engineering. Dr. Pellman, who had earlier stepped down as the chairman of the MTBI committee, remained a member of the committee representing the NFL. Dr. Casson, who had repeatedly denied any association between football and chronic brain damage, was also a member of the MTBI committee, as well as Dr. Viano, who coauthored the letter requesting the retraction of our first case report of gridiron dementia. As you may have noticed, no neuropathologist is a member of the committee, just like in 1994.

There were thirteen members of the retired player study committee, which included nine doctors, three PhDs, and one registered nurse. The doctors comprised three neuro-radiologists, one radiologist, three neurologists, one neurosurgeon, and one sports medicine physician. The PhDs comprised two in biomedical engineering and one in neuropsychology. Again Drs. Pellman, Casson, and Viano were members of this study group. Seven members who were on the MTBI committee of the NFL were also members of the study group commissioned to investigate retired football players, representing about 50 percent of both groups. Again, no neuropathologist or epidemiologist was in the study group investigating retired NFL players. My opinion regarding the NFL's May 22, 2007, press release was that the league was back to where it started in 1994, the same old way of doing things and the same old boys' club.

On July 14, 2004, after our first dementia case was confirmed in a retired NFL player, we sent a letter, and a follow-up letter a couple of months later, to a representative of the NFL Hall of Fame proposing a comprehensive, multifaceted, longitudinal study of every Hall of Famer over their remaining lifetimes and a possible examination of their brains when they died to determine the epidemiology of gridiron dementia in this representative cohort of retired NFL players. We had proposed that each Hall of Famer would visit Pittsburgh every six months for neuropsychiatric, neurological, and neuroradiological examinations and fol-low-up to monitor them for the development of dementia and major depression. Baseline genetic testing would be performed for every Hall of Famer at the beginning of the study to determine their genetic profiles. When they died, we would examine their brains for neuropathological evidence of gridiron dementia. This study would have involved all NFL Hall of Famers, who at the time numbered about 241. At the time this book was written, almost three years later, we have not heard from the NFL Hall of Fame. We never even received a courteous reply letter to acknowledge receipt of our letters and probably turn down our offer.

5

WHAT DO FOOTBALL PLAYERS KNOW ABOUT CONCUSSIONS?

Many amateur and professional football players have complained that organizers and governing agencies of all levels of football have not provided them with sufficient information and education regarding the dangers of concussions and the possible delayed effects of concussions derived from playing football. These complaints may be justified, because comprehensive programs for the education of football players at all levels of participation are essentially nonexistent. Players have argued that they should be made aware of the possible dangers of concussions before they begin playing football, and the judgment to play football should be made by each individual player after he has been fully informed of the pos-sible dangers of chronic brain damage caused by football.

Most professional football players are aware that blows and bangs to the head are incidental to the game. Many are aware of some consequences of such blows, including the occasional noises in the ears, transient alterations of aware-ness, visual symptoms and sensations of wooziness and fog-giness, dizziness, headaches, and loss of balance during or after a game. Ironically, while players frequently experience these symptoms, they rarely realize that they are suffering from the effects of repeated concussions. They simply dis-miss these symptoms as part of the game and do not link them to concussions. In fact, a majority of amateur and pro-fessional football players do not know what concussions are, and they do not know that repeated concussions may be very dangerous and can result in brain damage, dementia, and major depression later in life. Many players understand that repeated concussions could be harmful only when they are told so by their doctors in their middle and later years, when they are already suffering from early signs of demen-tia and from major depression. At this time, they cannot do anything about this realization, for it is already too late.

The number of concussions a football player may suf-fer may depend, to an extent, on the playing position. The players in American football who suffer the largest num-bers of concussions are offensive linemen, defensive line-men, linebackers, and defensive backs. Concussions can manifest as a variety of acute and delayed symptoms, which may be transient or persistent, lasting a couple of seconds to many weeks and months. Persistent postconcussion symptoms and signs may persist for years and may progress to a chronic traumatic encephalopathy. Symptoms and signs of concussions and the so-called postconcussion syndrome may include sensations of fogginess, sensations of haziness, dizziness, drowsiness, feeling slowed down, fatigue, headaches, nausea, vomiting, numbness, tingling sensations, ringing in the ears, loss of memory, or other memory problems, sensitivity to noise, sensitivity to light, trouble falling asleep, sadness, depression, nervousness, irritability, excess sleep, poor concentration, and poor balance. Unfortunately many players suffer from one or more of these symptoms during their careers and even decades after their retirement from football without having any remote suspicion that their symptoms may be the result of repeated concussions and subconcussions they sustained from the play of football.

Only 2 to 8 percent of all football players at the high school, college, and professional levels are diagnosed with concussions by team athletic trainers, coaches, and physicians. However, when players are anonymously surveyed retrospectively after the season, 15 to 70 percent of high school, college, and professional football players admit to suffering concussion symptoms during each season. Up to 70 percent of concussions suffered by football players may not be reported to the coach, trainers, or medical staff. This number is even greater when we add concussions suffered by players in practice and subconcussions suffered during practice and during games.

Concussions in football are obviously massively underreported, and several reasons account for this trend. The first reason is lack of education of players, coaches, and athletic trainers. Information about concussions is not made available to the players in a broad and well-organized manner. Consequently players do not know when they suffer concussions, do not know that they should report concussions to the coaches and team physicians, and do not know how concussions should be treated. The most common documented reasons why concussions may not be reported are that the injured players do not know when they suffer concussions and do not think concussions are serious enough to warrant medical attention. A secondary reason certainly is players feeling that by reporting their injuries, their playing time will be limited.

The father of a young professional football player once told me about a discussion he had with his son regarding concussions. His son had asked him if concussions were those times during a game one would feel dazed after a tackle and see stars. He had laughed and said that we thought too much, it was only part of the game; you feel dazed, medical staff comes to you to ask you one or two silly questions like your name and the date, you answer them, and that is it—you get back in the game. You may have headaches for a day or two, and you will get over it. As unbelievable as it may seem, this is the prevalent belief system in the culture of competitive football; concussions, even repeated concussions, are harmless. We know now that this belief system is misinformed.

Concussions, especially repeated concussions, are dangerous and can result in chronic brain damage. Due to poor education, misinformation, and massive underreporting of concussions, players are frequently returned to play when they should not be returned to play. Players with a prior history of loss of consciousness have a risk of loss of consciousness that is four times that of players without a prior history of loss of consciousness; over 70 percent of players who lose consciousness following a concussion are returned to play the same day.

Other very disturbing reasons that players do not report concussions are competitiveness and machismo. Football is a highly competitive sport, and over the years football players have developed a strong sense of masculine pride, which sometimes may border on exaggerated masculinity. It has become commonplace for football players, who are typically well-built and massive people, to possess an exaggerated and exhilarating sense of power and strength, which the advertising media sometimes take to mythical levels. It is believed, and is actually the pervasive subculture, that football players should not complain about the difficulties of playing football. Tough men do not cry. Placing your hands over your head and complaining about the effects of concussions are deemed as signs of weakness. A macho player should be able to play through concussions, and even the trainers and coaches support and perpetuate this misconception. This macho camaraderie among teammates discourages a player from reporting a concussion since such a report may cause him to be taken out of play. Many times players want to remain competitive, remain in the game, remain a significant part of the game plan, and be seen by other teammates as strong and tough by playing through concussions. The players may feel they are letting down their teammates if they report a concussion, since they are expected to ignore concussions

and stay on the playing field. The bottom line, however—
macho or not macho—is that players are afraid of being
sidelined, losing their starting positions, losing their roles
on the team, and even eventually losing their jobs with their
anticipated six-, seven-, or eight-figure salaries and bonuses.
Concussions or no concussions, show them the money and
they will play. The adverse consequences are that players
play through concussions, are not educated about concussions, care nothing about concussions, and even return to play many times in the same game after suffering
concussions.

The claim by the MTBI committee of the NFL that only
a minority of professional players suffer concussions may
not be true, for concussions are massively underreported.
Even with the small percentage of concussions reported by
players, 12 to 17 percent of players who suffer one to three
reported concussions are returned to play immediately.
Fifty to 60 percent of NFL players who suffer one to three
reported concussions are not removed from play, and about
60 percent of players with second reported concussions return to play within one day. These are alarming rates and
confirm the dangerous disregard in American football of
the deleterious effects of concussions to the brain. If this
high proportion of NFL players with reported concussions
play through their concussions and are not removed from
play, there would not be any motivation for players to report
their concussions, since it would likely make little or no difference whether they would be removed from play or not.
Rather than being perceived as weak, players would prefer
to keep on playing and not complain of concussions' signs

and symptoms. Since the majority of concussions and sub-concussions suffered by football players are not reported, it would not be conjectural to state that the culture in American football is for players to play through concussions and subconcussions. In fact, the MTBI committee of the NFL supports players remaining in the game after suffering a single concussion or repeated concussions. The committee members claim that players who are concussed and return to the same game have fewer signs and symptoms than those removed from play. They have asserted that return to play does not involve a significant risk of a second injury either in the same game or during the season. The MTBI committee of the NFL finds it appropriate and recommends that NFL team physicians immediately return players to the game after suffering concussions when the player has become asymptomatic. This stance is simply shocking.

6

DEPRESSION: NEUROLOGY AND FAMILY FACTORS

I have been asked repeatedly by members of the media during press interviews, and by my colleagues and fellow doctors during conferences, if playing football and repeated concussions from playing football can cause depression and suicide. My answer is yes. Do repeated concussions sustained from playing football cause depression and suicide in every person who plays football? My answer is no. As with boxers, I expect about 20 percent of football players to develop major depression and possibly suicidal behavior following repeated concussions. Currently we cannot predict who is at risk and who is not.

The definitive and confirmatory evidence for dementia, major depression, and suicide caused by playing football can only be provided by a complete autopsy with a neuropathologic examination of the brain. The microscopic study of the brain using a specific battery of antibodies can reveal the tissue evidence of gridiron dementia, major depression, and suicide. When the brain reveals the pathognomonic protein accumulations and conformations, a diagnosis of chronic traumatic encephalopathy or gridiron dementia can be rendered with a reasonable degree of medical certainty.

The brains of football players that I have examined revealed the accumulation of abnormal proteins called tau proteins, which form abnormal structures in the brain called neurofibrillary tangles and neuritic threads. These proteins and structures are typically found in a type of dementia called tangle-only dementia. This type of dementia predominantly occurs in patients in their eighties and nineties. It is rather an enigma that the brain of a football player in his forties should present like the brain of an eighty-year-old.

Another even more interesting factor in the association between football players and depression is that depression is a major biologic component of the majority of dementias. Since gridiron dementia is a type of dementia induced by repeated concussions, there is no justifiable reason to exclude major depression as a component of gridiron dementia. Not every depressed person commits suicide. Therefore, not every depressed football player with gridiron dementia will commit suicide.

Certain regions in the brain synthesize specific proteins (neurotransmitters) for the maintenance of mood and optimal happiness. The abnormal proteins that accumulate in gridiron dementia also accumulate in these regions of the brain that maintain mood and happiness. Over a prolonged period of time, these abnormal proteins alter the normal functioning of the mood centers and actually kill off the brain cells in these mood centers, resulting in mood disorders and depression.

Major depressive disorder is the disease most commonly associated with a completed suicide. Suicide is the major life-threatening complication of depression. About 66 percent of people who commit suicide suffer from a major depressive disorder. Approximately 7 percent of men and 1 percent of women who suffer from major depression will carry out a complete suicide. Football players who suffer from major depression associated with gridiron dementia may commit suicide. The risk of suicide in patients with a major depressive disorder is about twenty times that of the general population. This risk level is even higher in football players who suffer from gridiron dementia. Completed suicides in football players suffering from gridiron dementia constitute fatal outcomes of events that began with repeated concussions sustained from playing football.

Genetic analyses of a specific target gene in the first three NFL players we have examined revealed the presence of a specific gene allele in all three players. It is possible that a more comprehensive study, like the one we have proposed, may amplify this trend and identify the possible gene markers for football players who may possess an increased genetic risk for gridiron dementia and major depression. Such a study may also identify the possible role played by abuse of steroids in the development of gridiron dementia. (Personally, I doubt if steroids play any role in the development of gridiron dementia, because the majority of individuals who suffer chronic brain damage caused by trauma outside football do not abuse steroids.)

Like most other diseases, depression is a multifactorial disease with many causes, including biological, genetic, environmental, psychological, medical, and other causes. Simultaneous occurrence of more than one group of causes in one patient will generate an additive synergism that may result in an increased risk of developing depression, more severe forms of depression, or depression that is resistant to treatment. The cause of major depression in football players who suffer from gridiron dementia can be categorized under the biological causes of major depression. In this instance, as in other dementia patients, there is an identifiable and underlying biologic abnormality of the brain that is causally associated with the depression. For gridiron dementia to be determined as the major causal factor of major depression or suicide in a football player, direct tissue analysis and examination of the brain must be performed either via an autopsy or via a brain biopsy to identify the pathognomonic microstructural tissue abnormalities. The causal association will be buttressed and supported by a clinical symptomatology of dementia and major depression.

A more effective pharmacotherapy for depression associated with gridiron dementia may be drugs that clear or impede the accumulation of the abnormal proteins that are causing the dementia and depression. Popular antidepressants like Prozac, which enhance the effects of certain types of proteins (neurotransmitters) in the brain, may not be the most effective drug treatment modality for this type of depression.

A family history of depression may increase the risk of a child in that family developing depression. There is approximately an elevenfold increased risk of a child developing depression in a family with a clinical history of depression in a parent. The occurrence of gridiron dementia in a football player who possesses other risk factors for depression, or who possesses other causes of depression, is more likely to create a significant deleterious synergism that will potentiate the severity of the depression and increase the risk of eventual suicide. From every perspective one chooses to look at the global forensic scenario of major depressive illness, the tissue-confirmed presence of gridiron dementia will remain a significant and major independent contributory factor to the cumulative degree of depression and the occurrence of suicide attempts and completed suicides.

7

WHAT SHOULD WE DO?

Media response to the issues surrounding gridiron dementia has been amazing. I have been interviewed by over fifty media and professional organizations—local, national and even international newspapers, magazines, radio stations, television stations, Web sites, and scientific newsletters and journals—on the subject of dementia and depression in football players. Some flew to Pittsburgh for a face-to-face interview in front of a camera. These interviews taught me that people from all walks of life and every background have the same questions regarding football and concussions. Everyone yearns for answers to many questions, some out of curiosity, others out of legitimate fears for themselves, family, and friends.

I remember one interview very vividly. I had just returned home from work and was reviewing my mail for the day when my cell phone rang. It turned out to be the quiet and fearful voice of a middle-aged man who asked whether he could send his brain to me when he died since he was planning to commit suicide. I asked him why he would want to do that. He said he played football and suffered several concussions, and he had been suffering from what he called "mental disturbances," including major depression that his physicians had not been able to treat. I was stunned. I felt his pain. I experienced his trepidation just like the consternation of many other people who wrote and called me to share their stories of concussions, chronic headaches, and depression. At some points I felt so helpless. What should we all do?

Another interview also comes to mind. I was driving back to Pittsburgh around 6:00 p.m. when my cell phone rang. The caller was a North Carolina newspaper columnist who was completing an article that would be published the next day. He said he needed to speak with me immediately. I rarely turn down any requests made by members of the press, so I immediately exited the freeway, parked in a McDonald's parking lot, and spoke with him while the snow piled up outside my car. At the end of his fifteen-minute interview, he asked if I thought football was a dangerous sport. I paused and said that I would not answer that question. It was outside my area of competence and professional jurisdiction to make a judgment on whether football was a dangerous sport. I told him that his last question was a sociopolitical question that I could not and should not answer. He instantly redirected his question and asked me if I would let my son play football. My immediate response was no. He said thank you and hung up. I did not know if I did the right thing by answering "no" to his final question. I do not want to be dragged into sociopolitical and cultural debates about football. I am a scientist, not a sociologist or politician. But when I pulled back onto the freeway, I had a sense of peace and calm. At least I was convinced that when my son comes of age, I will not allow him to play football.

As citizens of a civilized nation, each individual can do something significant about these newly emerged concussion questions. We have the opportunity to change our perceptions about retired football players who seemingly cannot "make it" after retirement. Truthfully, many retired football players struggle socioeconomically after retirement and experience progressive decline from celebrity status to oblivion. Until we were given the opportunity in 2002, no one examined these players' brains after they died to determine the presence or absence of football-induced brain damage. Traditionally no one had thought about this earlier and no one had examined the brains of retired football players until we were put in the position of examining such a brain in 2002.

There is a reasonable scientific probability that many retired football players who are struggling socioeconomically, or who are manifesting psychological and behavioral abnormalities, may be suffering from gridiron dementia or concussion-drunk syndrome. We cannot quantify this reasonable probability until we look at the brains of every retired football player who dies. The only definitive way to confirm a diagnosis of gridiron dementia is to directly examine brain tissue, before or after death. It sounds very morbid, but the reality of life is that we all die someday.

This reality is also the reality of my profession as a forensic neuropathologist. In life, we can show these football players greater compassion, understanding, and support and be less critical of them. It may not, after all, be their fault. We should all come together to study this disease in a more systematic manner and probably come up with prophylactic and even therapeutic interventions.

Another question that arises frequently from parents is whether their sons should continue to play football in elementary, middle, and high schools. From a neuroscience perspective, we know that at birth the brain of a child is not fully developed. The brain of a child continues to develop and mature from birth until the late teenage years around the age of eighteen, when the brain assumes its peak development capacity. A very basic question is if it would be wise to subject a developing brain to repeated concussions and shearing, no matter how innocuous the concussions may seem. Remember, there is no safe concussion, just as there is no safe cigarette smoking. The responsibility of the judgment of allowing children to play football or not to play football is on the parents. My duty, and the duty of any expert, is to establish the scientific facts and to firmly educate people, not to make judgments and rulings. However, empirical scientific research has confirmed unquestionably that the developing brain of a child or a teenager is more vulnerable to the deleterious effects of all types of concussions than the developed adult brain. The brains of children and early teenagers are more likely to suffer adverse delayed outcomes of repeated concussions than the adult brain.

In another live television interview, again in a parking lot via my cell phone, a retired football player asked me if I thought that the current rigid helmets may be adding to the escalating problem of concussions. My answer was yes, they may be contributing to the effects of concussions sustained during the play of football. Wearing a helmet can give a player a false sense of confidence to tackle with his head, fall with his head, or even hit other players with his head, increasing the cumulative number of blows to the skull and the brain. The current helmet is designed to be rigid and nonpliant, to protect the head from impact biomechanical loading. The helmet has done a marvelous job in preventing fractures of the skull and brain hemorrhages. However, there may be room for improvement regarding inertial biomechanical loading and concussions of the brain. The current helmets may be redesigned to cushion the transference of shearing forces and energy to the brain and mitigate concussions of the brain. Given the advances in materials science, this possibility should be explored by biomechanical engineers. It is common sense and not wishful thinking that a more pliant and padded but firm helmet will reduce the amount of shearing forces that eventually reach the brain with or without impact.

In order to move forward on the issue of long-term football-induced brain damage, we have to establish a longitudinal, prospective, multi-institutional, and multidisciplinary study that will follow every NFL player from draft to death. There should be about four or five designated centers across the country where players visit annually or semiannually for a comprehensive medical examination that would include genetic testing, neuropsychiatric evaluation, neurological examination, and neuroradiologic examination. When the players die, their brains will have to be examined and sections conserved in a tissue bank for possible tissue studies in the future as technology evolves. Following the draft, the baseline clinical characteristics of each player should be established as a reference point.

The five centers should be university based and may include a center each in the Northwest, Southwest, Northeast, Southeast, and Midwest depending on what demographics are considered. Neuroradiologists, psychiatrists, psychologists, neurologists, neurosurgeons, neuropathologists, molecular biologists, and injury epidemiologists are the multidisciplinary specialists who should be involved in this study. It should be a long-term longitudinal study that should last at least one generation. Emerging results and trends may be published every five years. This study can be paid for by the NFL, the players (a very small percentage of each player's salary), the financial sponsors of the NFL, and grants/gifts from individuals, organizations, and corporations.

During and after such a long-term and prospective study, we can elucidate the underlying etiologies and cascades of this disease in view of identifying who is at risk and quantifying the risk. Once we better understand the biology of gridiron dementia, we can advance the research to identify ways that we can prevent it and even treat it. America is the most endowed country in the world, with the best minds and brains. As Bill Gates once said, if you gather the smartest minds in a room and present them with a problem, they can solve whatever problem you have. And as Bill Clinton once said, America is a country where you can be whatever you want to be as long as you are ready to work for it.

America, we *can* do it, so let us do it. Rather than debating and contesting the issue of concussions in football and apportioning blame, let us all come together and solve this national problem, for what would life be in America without football? Football is the soul of America.

PART TWO

The Lives and Fates of Three Football Players

8

MICHAEL "IRON MIKE" WEBSTER

Michael Lewis Webster was born in Tomahawk, Wisconsin, on March 18, 1952. He died at the ripe age of fifty years old on September 24, 2002, in Pittsburgh, Pennsylvania. Mike Webster was inducted into the Pro Football Hall of Fame in 1997, and in 1999 he was ranked by *Sporting News* magazine as the seventy-fifth-greatest football player who ever lived. Regrettably, Mike Webster paid a very expensive price for his brilliant career and accomplishments in professional football. Mike was perceptibly mentally disabled by the time he retired from the NFL in 1990. He suffered from dementia and major depression. Following his retirement from the NFL, some people who knew him and who couldn't understand what was going on with Mike prejudged him to be going crazy.

Mike grew up on a potato farm near Tomahawk, Wisconsin, in a dysfunctional family. His parents divorced when he was only ten years old, and both parents were alcoholics. Mike's younger brother later served time in jail for a sex-related offense. His father was an overbearing disciplinarian who probably subjected Mike to episodes of physical abuse.

In high school Mike woke up early in the morning to complete his farm chores before riding the school bus to his rural school, which was eighteen miles from home. His obligations to his father's farm and a dependency on the bus made it impossible for him early in high school to participate in football practices, but he still was a Green Bay Packers fan. He began playing football in his junior year of high school only when his high school football coach volunteered to personally drive Mike to and from school and made it possible for him to stay late for practice and still do his farm chores.

He played well enough in high school to earn a football scholarship to the University of Wisconsin, where he had a brilliant college football career. He was a lineman, his team's most valuable player, and was named as center for the All-Big-Ten team. He was a three-year starter and honor student at Wisconsin and was drafted by the Pittsburgh Steelers in the fifth round of the 1974 NFL draft.

Mike served as backup center and guard for the Steelers for two years. In his third year of professional football in 1976, he became the starting center, after which his career soared. Mike Webster was so tough and durable that he was nicknamed "Iron Mike." He was considered to be the strongest Steelers player and won the Ironman Competition in 1980. During his time, he was purported to be the strongest NFL player. His work ethic was impeccable. He was diligent in a vicious fashion.

Mike did not consider himself to be a great athlete, and he had low self-esteem. He believed that to remain competitive he had to work much harder in training and practice than most other players. In college, Mike weighed only 225 pounds and measured six feet, two inches tall. This was a relatively small body frame by NFL standards. Mike had to do something about his body when he was drafted into the league. He lifted weights, built his body, gained weight, and even exhibited evidence of the use of anabolic steroids, which were not yet banned by the NFL. He turned himself into an intimidating 260-pounder.

His accomplishments in the NFL speak for themselves. He played for the Pittsburgh Steelers from 1974 to 1988 and for the Kansas City Chiefs in 1989 and 1990. He was the offensive captain of the Pittsburgh Steelers for nine seasons. The Steelers won the Super Bowl four times within six seasons from 1975 to 1980, and Mike was a member of the Steelers teams that won those Super Bowls, serving as the captain of three of these championship teams. Mike Webster was the last of the twenty-two Steelers players who played on all four Super Bowl championship winning teams to leave the Steelers. By the time he retired in 1990, he had played in the NFL for seventeen seasons and had played in 245 games. He was known to refuse to leave the lineup even for serious injuries. Between 1976 and 1985, over ten seasons, Mike Webster played in 177 consecutive games and was in the starting lineup in 150 consecutive games. He played in nineteen playoff games and six AFC championship games, in addition to the four Super Bowls. He was honored as All-AFC five times, All-Pro seven times, and played in the Pro Bowl nine times (1979 to 1986, 1988), the first five as a starter. He was honored as a member of the All-Time NFL team in 2000, as a member of the NFL Seventy-Fifth Anniversary All-Time team, as a member of the NFL's 1980s' and 1970s' All-Decade Teams. Simply put, he was one of the NFL's best linemen ever. By every yardstick, he had an overachieving professional football career. However, he also admitted to using anabolic steroids at different points in his career.

Mike Webster was nothing but an invincible and brilliant player. He epitomized every sense of the tough and versatile veteran. But what happened to Iron Mike after his retirement can only be fathomed by the deeply intuitive and curious mind. The tough man was reduced to a demented, paranoid, depressed, and defenseless man by no fault of his own. The hardest part was the effect on his family, his wife and four children, who painfully watched him as he progressively deteriorated. One memorable day after dinner, in the presence of friends and family, Mike opened the oven in the kitchen, unzipped his pants, urinated into the oven, closed it, and walked away, believing in his mind that he had just used the toilet to relieve himself. As painful and embarrassing as it may have been to the family and close friends, in Mike's frail and degenerating mind the oven had become a commode.

Barely a year after his retirement in 1990, Iron Mike was visibly perturbed mentally and cognitively. Over a period of six years after his retirement, Mike lost all his estimated assets of $2 million to $3 million due to grossly diminished cognitive and executive functioning. He made poor business decisions and investments. He passed on great job offers and opportunities. At some point after his retirement from the NFL he had over eight jobs within a four-year span. He either began, or was part of, many start-up ventures, which all failed. Lawsuits followed his business failures, and his annuities and investments were all seized as collateral for the bank loans, which remained unpaid. At the end Mike had opened over sixty-five checking accounts and safe-deposit boxes in Pennsylvania, Arkansas, West Virginia, and Wisconsin. He simply drifted downhill socioeconomically.

Just about eighteen months after Mike moved his family into a large Victorian house that he had purchased, the bank foreclosed. Mike was known to leave his home, his wife, and his children for days at a time, for no just cause. Nobody seemed to understand why. His loving wife unknowingly presumed that Mike was mad at her and that was what made him desert the family when he left their home. Pam did not realize that her poor husband may have been suffering from the effects of a brain that had been damaged by repeated blows to the head while playing football.

Mike Webster was married to his wife, Pam, for eighteen years. They met on a blind date in college. Pam had noticed that something was wrong with Mike in his final five seasons in the NFL. Whatever it was, it was slow but progressive. Mike was gradually losing control of his mind with spontaneous anger episodes, personality changes, disorientation, and loss of memory. They separated in 1992, two years after Mike retired from the NFL, and finally divorced six months before Mike died in 2002. This divorce has been Pam's biggest regret. But it was not her fault, for she did not understand that football had taken the best of Mike Webster.

Was Mike Webster one of the many professional football players whom society may have wrongfully presumed to be dim-witted, brainless, and unintelligent, and who could not excel in life after or outside football? Or was he really a victim of his circumstances? Was Mike Webster, having received concussions in his career, victimized by the delayed sequelae of playing professional football—delayed sequelae that had remained unrecognized? A conservative estimate may indicate that Mike Webster endured over twenty thousand violent collisions while he played professional football in practice and in regular season, playoff, and Super Bowl games. Yet Mike Webster was not specifically treated for concussions by his team physicians. In the 1970s and 1980s, we did not know so much about concussions and about the effects of concussions sustained from playing football. Apparently Mike may not have complained of symptoms of concussions, or he may have complained and those complaints may not have been associated with concussions. We now know better.

Mike Webster became homeless. Day after day, night after night, he huddled cold and alone on the floors of the Amtrak railway station he called home in downtown Pittsburgh. What an ironic outcome for a man who had won four Super Bowl rings in six seasons. Unfortunately, on his way to four Super Bowl rings, he had received thousands of hits on his head and suffered many concussions. Mike's brain had apparently given up on him. He lived on potato chips and dry cereal, possibly handed to him by passersby. Sometimes he even forgot to eat for days. He paid less and less attention to what he ate and how he looked. He did not, however, give up on his steady flow of Coca-Cola, caffeine, and nicotine. At some point his weight dropped by thirty-five pounds. Sometimes he slept in his beat-up pickup truck, which had a garbage bag duct-taped over a missing window.

Sometimes he seemed not to care, glassy-eyed, staring into space. He drifted into a vagabond life between Kansas City, Pittsburgh, Philadelphia, rural West Virginia, and Wisconsin. When he became tired he would sometimes park his beat-up truck wherever convenient—in a parking lot at the airport, bus station, train depot, grocery store, or strip mall—and catch some much-needed sleep. When he had the cash he would sleep in a cheap roadside motel. He lived in despair and hopelessness. He contemplated suicide but held himself back because God would not want him to kill himself and he would not be able to help his family if he were dead.

On one of his son's birthdays, Mike Webster did not show up for the party. He lay alone in a dark room, in a cheap motel, intoxicated with painkillers and sedatives, with a bucket of vomit by his bed. Mike could not help it since he was taking a myriad of medications. Just a few of his medications included Prozac, Zoloft, or Paxil for depression; Ritalin or Dexedrine to keep him mentally alert; narcotic and nonnarcotic painkillers in various combinations (Tramadol, Propoxyphene, Hydrocodone) to ward off pain; benzodiazepines to prevent panic attacks and anxiety; Selegiline to minimize movement disorders; and so many other drugs. Unfortunately, most of these drugs act on the brain and manifest combined synergistic depressive effects. Any individual taking a combination of these drugs would remain bed-bound on his son's birthday.

Mike desperately needed all these drugs. His head throbbed constantly, his hearing was going bad, his spine hurt badly from herniated discs, his damaged right ankle hurt badly and caused him to limp, his right shoulder hurt badly from torn ligaments, his right elbow hurt badly from a dislocation, his knees were almost destroyed from years of tough play and grinding, his knuckles and joints of his fingers were swollen and deviated from seventeen years of hard play in the NFL. Mike had simply lost control of his body to the injuries sustained from playing football. He needed his painkillers badly. At some points he even stunned himself repeatedly with a Taser gun in search of a few moments of peace from pain. Sometimes he inhaled vapors of ammonia to stay calm.

Yet the NFL denied him disability entitlements. A representative of the NFL once contended that although Mike ran several businesses that ultimately failed, he was not entitled to permanent disability benefits simply because his businesses did not succeed. Poor, anguished Mike was known on different occasions to have placed rambling calls to friends and family asking for his way home. He once said apologetically to a friend whom he called for directions, "All I see is trees . . . ."

In one of the apartments Mike had rented during his postretirement quagmire, his seventeen-year-old son had placed a flag on the front window to enable Mike to identify their apartment. Still Mike sometimes found himself knocking hard on a neighbor's door late at night when the key would not fit. He probably did not figure out that if the key did not fit, then it was probably the wrong door and the wrong apartment. He did not remember to watch out for the flag on the front window.

As the years went slowly by, Mike was known to have locked himself up on many occasions, curled up in a fetal position for three or four days, thinking of life and contemplating suicide. He even kept personal journals that were so convoluted and confusing that even Mike himself, in his lucid moments, did not comprehend them. For about ten days every month, Mike's mental functioning improved slightly. During these times he wept when he read his distorted journals, which he couldn't even remember writing. Sometimes he remembered first and last names of transient acquaintances in the remote past; other times he wouldn't remember that it was winter, and he would walk into the frigid morning weather with only a shirt. Other times in ten-degree Fahrenheit weather, Mike complained that he felt too hot.

Mike progressively became paranoid. He avoided restaurants and other public places because he believed some people were out to get him. He believed that people were plotting a conspiracy against him. He dealt only in cash so that no one would be able to track his dealings. He would wake up at night around 2:00 to 3:00 a.m. to go shopping at Wal-Mart. He even wrote a letter once to George H. W. Bush to tell the U.S. president about the conspiracy against Mike Webster. He became increasingly violent and exhibited fluctuating moods with episodes of unjustifiable anger and agitation. He became verbally abusive to close family and friends. He would beat up cars and trucks with baseball bats during some periods of agitation, breaking windows and headlamps.

Mike consulted many physicians in his post-NFL life journey. Mike was tagged with a myriad of diagnoses, which included major depression and so-called postconcussion syndrome. Postconcussion syndrome is one of the many diagnoses that some doctors use when they truly do not understand what is happening. But this diagnosis became extremely useful after Mike Webster's death. That phrase, postconcussion syndrome, brought us to where we are today. In fact, I am writing this book today because of this phrase, another act of serendipity since I never knew Mike Webster until after he died.

After his death in Pittsburgh, Pennsylvania, an unspecified physician listed this nonspecific phrase in Mike Webster's death certificate as a factor contributing to his demise. Through the act of divine providence, I was scheduled to perform autopsies at my office on the weekend of September 28, 2002. I had just completed fellowship training in neuropathology, so my brain was still full of academic stuff that I knew very well. I woke up that morning to prepare for work, and just before I left I turned on the television to listen to the morning talk shows. All over the channels was this talk about Mike Webster, a retired NFL player who had passed away on September 24, 2002, at the young age of fifty. All the television talk shows were pretty much making not-so-encouraging comments about this retired NFL player who was very competitive on football's field of play but was not the least bit competitive on the playing field of life. He was yet another professional athlete who failed woefully in business, who died broke, and who had been homeless. Luckily he did not commit suicide, but he did attempt suicide after retirement from the NFL.

In a way, my professional sense of decency as a neuropathologist was offended by what I heard on television about Mike Webster. I became angry for no reason. I felt the urge to do something, but what could I do? While I drove to work I contemplated how the television commentators might have known that Mike Webster could have been a victim of a disease similar to dementia pugilistica, or punch-drunk syndrome, which affected retired boxers. He played football for a long time; football is a high-impact contact sport, and he could have received so many blows to his head just as a boxer would have. But I saw myself as an insignificant doctor who had no clout, so I thought that my opinion would make no difference. I shrugged off the commentary and dismissed it as one of those injustices of life and moved on.

Little did I know that less than thirty minutes later I would meet Mike Webster in person, and in death he would call on my background and training to prove to the world that even unto death he was the tough and versatile Iron Mike. He was the competitive Mike that we had known him to be. He had another chance to prove the world wrong.

Death had liberated him from the shackles of his degenerated brain. This time around, repeated concussions, dementia, and major depression would not stop him. In death, Mike Webster compelled us all to remember that concussions sustained from playing football may be dangerous and can turn a tough man into a vegetable.

When I arrived at work in the late morning of Saturday, September 28, 2002, the embalmed body of Mike Webster was lying in the autopsy suite. Postconcussion syndrome, listed as a contributory factor to his death, is not a natural disease and would thus make the manner of his death accidental. Every accidental manner of death falls under the jurisdiction of the medical examiner. My office assumed jurisdiction of his death; the coroner requested a complete autopsy, which I had to perform. Being a neuropathologist, I was extremely interested in Mike's brain. Amazingly his brain appeared completely normal to the naked eye, but I was not fooled. I knew better. I saved his brain in formalin, a chemical that preserves human tissues and prevents the brain from decaying. Microscopic examination of his brain confirmed those thoughts I had in my car while I drove to work that morning of September 28, 2002.

I have always regarded forensic pathologists as advocates for the dead. We defend and speak for the dead. Our long years of education simply teach us the language of the dead. We learn to listen to them, and we hear the dead when they speak. We are the link between the dead and the living. Many times we can take what we learn from the dead and apply it to the living to save lives, understand our lives better, and improve the quality of our lives. Forensic pathology therefore can be a very vital public health and safety tool if applied and translated appropriately and optimally. The dead speak to us through the means of evidentiary autopsy findings, tissue findings, patterns of trauma, and patterns of disease. The responsibility of the forensic pathologist is to identify these findings and patterns, interpret them, and translate them into the language of the living. We did exactly that with Mike Webster.

Mike Webster spoke to us through the patterns of disease in his tissues. We listened, heard him, and translated what he said to us. He said to us that it was not his fault. He said to us that he suffered from the effects of more than twenty thousand blows to his head while he played football. He told us to do something so that younger players who will come after him will not end up like him. He told us to be more compassionate, more understanding, and more patient with his peers who may already be suffering from what he endured.

Mike Webster's brain revealed the tissue substrates of gridiron dementia or football-induced chronic traumatic encephalopathy (CTE). Autopsy unquestionably confirmed that Mike Webster was a victim of repeated brain concussions sustained while playing football. His mental and psychosocial profiles and behavior after retirement from the NFL, including dementia and major depression were all due to an organic brain disease that playing football caused. While we had known about the existence of this disease in boxers for so many years, we did not realize that football players who seemingly did not sustain documented career-ending concussions may suffer from football-induced dementia and depression.

The case of Mike Webster was finally reported and published as a peer-reviewed scientific paper in the journal *Neurosurgery* in 2005. It was the very first reported and published case of autopsy-confirmed gridiron dementia in a retired NFL player in the history of medicine. Initially many people did not believe us, but after the case was published and presented in professional meetings across the country, and after we reported the second and third autopsy-confirmed cases, the doubting Thomases repented and became liberated into the light of the scientific truth. These case led to a major shift in scientific thought in the way we think about and study concussions in sports. In my opinion, in death, Mike Webster scored a final winning touchdown and won his fifth championship ring.

In his enshrinement speech in 1997, when he was elected into the Pro Football Hall of Fame, Mike rambled and digressed often, but he still made it through. Ironically he said in part that "you only fail if you don't finish the game. . . . Sometimes you can be down and struggling but as long as you keep working at it, you win. The important thing is that I'm here and moving forward." And yes, he moved forward even unto death. He was a winner in the true sense of the word.

After a prolonged fight by Mike Webster and his family, the NFL finally awarded him, in 1999, an annual disability benefit of over one hundred thousand dollars, which he received in the last three years of his life. Posthumously, in December 2004, his estate was awarded over three hundred thousand dollars to cover his disability payment for three years from 1996 to 1999. As a last resort, Mike Webster's wife and children sued the NFL Player Retirement Plan in the U.S. District Court of the Northern District of Maryland, asking for the NFL to rightfully push back Mike's legal disability date to the time he retired from the NFL. As pitiful as it may sound, a federal judge had to order the NFL benefits plan to pay Mike's family a maximum of $1.6 million in owed benefits, accrued interest, and fees, to which Mike was justifiably entitled. Still, the NFL appealed the ruling. Thankfully, the U.S. Court of Appeals for the Fourth Circuit in Richmond, Virginia, affirmed the lower court's ruling. This precedent meant, in effect, that the NFL retirement plan must pay disabled players the over $1 billion in benefits reserved for players who became disabled playing football in the NFL.

9

TERRY "T-BONE" LONG

Terrence (Terry) Luther Long was born in Columbia, South Carolina, on July 21, 1959. He unfortunately died at the young age of forty-five as a result of suicide. A completed suicide may be defined as an intentional or volitional, and premeditated, act to terminate one's life. Terry's suicidal act may not have been volitional. His suicide may have been invoked by the thoughts of a markedly diseased brain that was generating abnormal and extremely exaggerated responses to the daily stresses of life.

Terry's autopsy confirmed that football had stolen his brain from him. He was the second-ever-reported autopsy-proven case of gridiron dementia. His brain revealed changes that are found in the brains of elderly individuals who are suffering from some types of dementia. A good number of his brain cells were dead and gone. Many regions in the brain, including regions responsible for emotions and mood, showed large accumulations of abnormal proteins. No wonder Terry made several unsuccessful suicide attempts during and after the time he spent in the NFL. On June 7, 2005, he was compelled by the abnormal functioning of his brain to fatally overdose on antifreeze (ethylene glycol). This final and terminal act of suicide was the end stage of an advanced disease whose cascade was initiated by the very first blow to the head that Terry sustained while he played football as a teenager. Drinking antifreeze was the idea of a lunatic mind at work—a lunacy caused by a noncongenital disease, acquired from playing football.

Terry grew up a smart and shy kid. He was extremely caring and giving. Baptized at an early age at the Ridgewood Baptist Church in Columbia, South Carolina, he was raised in a Christian family. As he grew older he became religious, and as an adult he professed Jesus as his Lord and savior. Terry attended high school from 1973 to 1977. He began working as a mason's apprentice in his first year of high school and proved to be a very hard worker. He quickly learned the trade of bricklaying at this relatively tender age. Being a kindhearted and compassionate person, Terry began contributing at this young age to the upkeep of his entire family. His father had died suddenly when Terry was only a teenager. He chipped in the income he made from bricklaying to supplement his mother's meager wages. Terry was simply selfless and would not hesitate to deny himself to help another soul who may have been in need. He grew up to become a gentleman in the true sense of the word.

Immediately after high school, Terry enlisted in the
U.S. Armed Forces in 1977 and served in the Special Forces
Division until 1979. While in the army he continued to care
for his family and was blessed to discover his talent and
prowess in competitive sports. He participated in weight
lifting and football in the military. He quickly ascended the
football ranks in the military as an offensive tackle. It did
not take too long for everyone to recognize Terry as a budding football star. Ironically Terry was not an ardent fan of
having a military career, but he loved playing football in the
military. Luckily for him, he was recruited from the military
by football scouts in 1979 and attended Columbia Junior
College in South Carolina, where he earned fifteen credits
toward a degree in business administration. In college, his
reputation soared. As his coaches in the military predicted,
his fame rose quickly. College football scouts recognized a
premium football player. He was enticed with a full football
scholarship to transfer to another college.

Terry transferred from Columbia Junior College to East
Carolina University, where he was the starting offensive line
tackle from 1980 to 1984. He earned credits toward a bachelor's degree in physical education. Terry began to shine
like a star. A shining beam from heaven had lit his path.
Interestingly, Terry lifted weights while he played football
at East Carolina University, and he performed exceedingly
well in weight lifting. He was a tough and versatile athlete
who measured just under six feet tall, but he weighed 284
pounds. He received many accolades and set many records
in college. At one point he was voted the third-strongest
power lifter in the world. He had the best power-lifting

records in North Carolina, when he could hoist 2,203 pounds in a squat, bench press, and dead lift. At another point in 1983 he was considered the strongest college football player in the United States. He was a college All-American guard, and as he entered his senior year, Terry won the Walter Camp Football Foundation All-American Award and the Janet Overton Memorial Award for the most outstanding senior.

Terry was drafted into the NFL in the fourth round of the 1984 draft by the Pittsburgh Steelers as a right guard. He started the Steelers' 1984 season opener as left guard for an injured player. He remained a fixture in the lineup and moved to starting right guard. Terry was an essential part of the Steelers' offense, which was routinely ranked among the NFL's best in the mid-1980s at preventing sacks. Terry played for eight consecutive years with the Steelers, from 1984 to 1992, alongside many great NFL players, including Mike Webster. Terry exhibited an admirable camaraderie with his team owners, coach, and fellow players. He was simply loved by everyone and developed very strong friendships with members of his team and other NFL teams. He was fondly nicknamed "T-Bone." Because of his extremely affable personality, people naturally gravitated toward him. In 1989 Terry became the first East Carolina University player to donate a football scholarship to his alma mater. He was one of the few Steelers players who were profiled on a youth trading card sponsored in part by local police departments.

In the winter of 1990, while Terry was recovering from knee surgery, he experimented with over-the-counter medications like yohimbe bark, ginseng root, and various muscle-building proteins. At the start of a training camp in July 1991, he was informed by his coach that his testosterone level was three times the NFL threshold. He was suspended by the NFL for four weeks without pay. Terry cried and suffered a reactive depression the day he heard the news of his positive steroid test on July 23, 1991. He attempted suicide the next day, brandishing a gun and threatening to shoot himself. He later swallowed a combination of sleeping pills and rat poison. He was taken to a local hospital, where he was treated and survived. He spent one week in the hospital and received psychological counseling. When he was released from the hospital, he started three games as left guard for the Steelers before he tore a muscle in his right arm. In early 1992 Terry's football career ended unexpectedly. The Steelers' new coach did not renew Terry's contract. Apparently Terry did not get along with the new coach.

Terry suffered at least one documented episode of a severe brain concussion, which was sustained during a game with the Houston Oilers in 1987. He suffered a head-on hit with an Oilers player and became lightheaded, dizzy, and confused. He was hospitalized overnight and discharged, although he still complained of lightheadedness, unsteadiness, and difficulty concentrating for several days. Ironically, to the naked eye he appeared physically fit and fine. Terry was taken out of play for only one week. In late 1990 Terry was involved in a motor vehicle accident in which the sport utility vehicle he was driving rolled over when he swerved to avoid hitting a deer. He experienced a brief loss of consciousness at the scene but recovered completely and was able to recall everything that transpired.

Like many of his peers in professional football, Terry Long sustained multiple injuries during his career in football. On many occasions, Terry privately admitted to his second wife, Lynne Long, that he sustained blows to his head numerous times while he played football. This normal and expected occurrence for football players was nothing to worry about, he said. He had at least four surgeries on his elbow, shoulder, and knee joints. Following his retirement from the NFL he developed a chronic infection of a sinus tract from retained surgical suture material, which had eroded one of his bones. After his retirement, Terry filed a workers' compensation claim with the NFL Players Association for chronic pain and stiffness in his shoulder and knee joints, which was obviously denied. As his retirement years rolled by, Terry's colleagues and friends thought him to be boyishly quiet and pleasant. His wife, Lynne, thought differently since she was close enough to Terry for her to notice what other people did not see. Terry was increasingly becoming a very scared and fearful man. He was becoming extremely paranoid. Many times in public gatherings and settings Terry would sweat profusely and uncontrollably for no reason. Sometimes he became extremely agitated when he was approached by people in public. Other times, he seemed very cool, calm, and collected. At these times, he would present an appropriately confident, successful, determined, and fun-loving demeanor.

Lynne met Terry in 1993 when Terry stopped by a nursing home to market the products of his produce company. Lynne worked as an administrator in the nursing home. At this time Terry was already very depressed. His neediness and boyish nature were actually what attracted Lynne to Terry. Terry literally broke down sobbing on several occasions when he visited Lynne's office, recounting how the NFL had let him down. He was hurting very deeply. Lynne and Terry began dating soon after they met, became engaged in 1993, and married in 1997. Terry had married his first wife around 1980 while he was in college. The marriage ended in a divorce. Terry's second marriage to Lynne, as one might expect, was a bumpy one. Lynne and Terry separated on and off beginning in 2000. Lynne finally moved into a new apartment in 2002. Lynne feared for her safety due to Terry's compulsive and irrational behavior, which oscillated from kind and gentle to aggressive and hostile. When Terry died in 2005, they were still legally married but separated.

According to Lynne, Terry exhibited totally new personas in their private life. Living with Terry became like riding a roller coaster with constant, spontaneous ups and downs without any warnings. Terry would often resort to a reclusive life and seclude himself from personal and social interactions with everyone, including family and friends. He would lock himself up in his house for a day or two and would not talk to anyone. Suddenly he would become exuberantly sociable again, seeking companionship and contact as if nothing had happened.

Terry had quite a bit of an entrepreneurial and industrious streak in him. While he played football for the Steelers he began a sole proprietorship company in 1988, four years before he stopped playing in the NFL. Supposedly this sole proprietorship lasted for only four years. During the life of this company, it was not unusual to find Terry awake in the early hours of the morning, sometimes as early as 3:00 a.m., distributing and filling his clients' orders around southwestern Pennsylvania. After his retirement from the NFL in 1992, he worked as a sales manager for another company, and one year later he formed his second corporation, a wholesale produce company. Some people characterized his business concepts as extraordinarily ambitious and risky, if not impractical. But he was a good salesman because of his magnetically charming personality. When he spoke, people listened, for he was believed to be a wealthy retired professional football player and a celebrity.

Yet again, in 1994, one year after he began his second company, Terry diversified his wholesale produce business and expanded into food processing and manufacturing. He formed a third corporation, which was a produce processing and manufacturing business that served local grocery chains. As his business expanded, Terry's problems in his personal and private life began to encroach on his business dealings and transactions. His skills and acumen in business management went up and down like a roller coaster, just as his moods did. Sometimes he was extremely hard working and highly driven; then suddenly, for no just cause, he would transgress into episodes of agitation and irritability that were not founded upon any tangible issues. At these times, Terry would become highly emotional and lose his ability to concentrate and focus on his business transactions and decision-making processes. There were extremes of highs and lows in his moods. Sometimes he would be very happy and buoyant, and suddenly he would become sullen and depressed. Consequently his businesses began to falter.

Unfortunately, his wife, who apparently did not understand what was going on with Terry, assumed that he had a manic-depressive personality. She thought complex rational thought was not one of Terry's strengths, for whenever she had asked him questions on complex subjects, Terry would dodge her questions and tell her that he would get back to her later.

The situation grew worse. Terry became more and more paranoid. He increasingly became untrusting of his business colleagues and partners. He became more controlling of his business subordinates and activities. The most damaging emergent traits for his businesses were his increasing impulsivity and his diminishing capacity to restrain himself. He would impulsively enter into contractual agreements and initiate deals without much thought, analysis, or research. His expected and projected revenue streams from these impulsive transactions never materialized. His businesses were suffering, and his coffers were shrinking although his altruistic nature remained intact. Despite his declining business performance, Terry still offered jobs to poor, young, inner-city men and women who needed someone to give them a second chance in life. In search of money and self-actualization himself, Terry desperately had to bail himself out one way or the other.

In 2000, Terry expanded his food service business into poultry and potato processing and packaging. He purchased a big poultry processing plant. It was only a matter of time before Terry's businesses would collapse financially. In 2003, he filed Chapter 11 bankruptcy for Terry Long Enterprises. The same day he filed for bankruptcy, his chicken processing plant was gutted by a fire. Terry Long was indicted on March 29, 2005, on federal charges of arson and mail fraud stemming from this fire. He was charged with setting fire to his plant for $1.1 million in insurance money and defrauding the state of nearly $1.2 million in business loans. Another unrelated warrant was held for Terry by authorities in Kansas City, Missouri, on a felony charge of writing bad checks.

Before his plant was gutted, Terry had found himself in a financial crisis. His behavior became more erratic, and he began to lose his social inhibitions, constraints, and etiquette. Finally, he intuited that something might be mentally wrong with him since he was even losing his ability to engage in routine activities of daily living. He voluntarily consulted a psychiatrist who diagnosed him with major depressive disorder. It may have been already too late, since Terry had constant suicidal ideations and had started verbalizing thoughts of suicide. He actually made several suicide attempts with prescription drugs and antifreeze. He was admitted several times to a psychiatric hospital for inpatient treatment. He attempted another suicide after his indictment by drinking antifreeze, and he had to be admitted via the emergency room into a local hospital where he was treated accordingly.

On June 7, 2005, a few weeks after his last discharge from the hospital for a suicide attempt, following his federal indictment, Terry was found in the morning lying on a couch at his home with an altered mental status. He was transported to a local hospital where he died several hours later. Laboratory analyses of his blood and urine samples indicated a fatal ingestion of ethylene glycol. Since his death was suspected to be a suicide, it fell under the jurisdiction of the county coroner, who ordered a full autopsy on the body of Terry Long. After his death, his wife, Lynne, said, "Terry's life was a road traveled up a tremendously successful hill and then unfortunately and suddenly down a rumbling, treacherous steep hill that was, I am now aware, beyond his ability to control." No statement could better describe Terry Long's life.

Terry Long arrived at my work bench, as had Mike Webster. Like Iron Mike's, Terry's brain looked normal to the naked eye. And as with Iron Mike, I saved the brain and fixed it in formalin for neuropathologic examination two weeks later. The brain that is not fixed in formalin has an extremely soft consistency and cannot be processed for microscopic examination. It takes approximately two weeks of complete submersion in formalin for the brain to become sufficiently hard for optimal tissue processing. Terry's autopsy confirmed that he overdosed on ethylene glycol, an odorless, colorless liquid with a sweet taste. Terry's brain developed acute chemical meningitis (inflammation of the coverings of the brain) due to the toxic effects of ethylene glycol. The autopsy also showed that one artery supplying his heart was moderately occluded by cholesterol plaques.

Additional microscopic examination and analysis of Terry's brain confirmed the presence of gridiron dementia. There were large accumulations of abnormal proteins (tau protein) in tissues and cells throughout his brain. A significant number of his brain cells had died and disappeared due to toxic effects of these proteins. Regions of his brain responsible for mood, emotions, and executive functioning were all damaged by accumulated abnormal proteins. These tissue changes were most probably responsible for his progressive neuropsychiatric symptoms and poor performance in business.

When Terry's autopsy diagnosis was released to the press, the reactions we received from some prominent and very accomplished NFL physicians were not in the least bit encouraging. In fact, some of the comments these physicians made were disparaging, condescending, insulting, and sometimes even conflicting. Some of their statements to the press were as follows:

> "That kind of injury [concussions] is something that happens in the NFL on a weekly basis."
> "To say he was killed by football, it's just not right, it's not appropriate."
> "I think it's not appropriate science when you have a history of no significant head injuries."
> "I think the conclusions drawn here are preposterous and a misinterpretation of facts."
> "I think it's fallacious reasoning, and I don't think it's plausible at all."
> "To go back and say that he was depressed from playing in the NFL and that led to his death fourteen years later, I think is purely speculative."

I was frightened but not intimidated. I kept the faith. I strongly believed that, if these doctors or the NFL came after me, the spirits of Mike Webster and Terry Long would shield me from any harm. "We" were all in search of the truth. We should not be afraid. With God on our side, we had nothing to fear. And, of course, I believed the Almighty was on our side. The case of Terry Long was exactly what was needed to quiet the skeptics. If the first case of autopsy-confirmed gridiron dementia (Mike Webster) was a chance occurrence or an aberration of the fundamental theories of probability, a second case was less likely to be. As expected, many more people, including some doctors who were associated with the NFL, began to have a change of heart and open up their ears, hearts, and minds to the message of these two football players. The association of dementia and major depression in contact-sport athletes was nothing new. However, dementia and major depression in football players due to repeated concussions sustained from playing football was something novel. It was just something nobody had thought about for so long.

The case of Terry Long was eventually published in the journal *Neurosurgery* in November 2006. It was also presented in several national meetings of professional medical associations across the United States. The resistance and scrutiny we faced this time around during the peer review of the paper for publication was much less than the first time around with the Mike Webster case. My very best day since this quagmire began was the day that Dr. Julian Bailes, one of the most prominent sports neurosurgeons in the world and someone whom I had not known, sought out my personal phone number and called me privately. He said things to me that were kind and extremely encouraging. In fact, he recognized the "good job" I was doing and said I should keep up the good work and not be distracted by the critics, no matter their constituency. I was truly rejuvenated by his comment. I remain very grateful to him, for at that time my spirit was almost at the point of being broken by the negativity in the press and by the response of the NFL physicians.

Terry's death did not receive the same spread and depth of press coverage as Mike Webster's. Mike may have been a more prominent NFL player since he was an NFL Hall of Famer. Mike's life after retirement may have been lived more in the public domain than Terry's. These may be seemingly obvious reasons, but there may be underlying cryptic reasons that these two individuals who suffered from the same disease received different responses from the public. These reasons may concern the terminal circumstances of their deaths. While Mike Webster attempted suicide, he never completed one. He eventually died of a heart attack. Terry Long attempted suicide several times, and unfortunately he completed his final suicide attempt.

The general populace across most cultures does not empathize or sympathize with our brothers and sisters who suffer from psychiatric diseases as they would empathize or sympathize with those of us who suffer from physical debilities and disabilities. A certain stigma is attached to suicide regarding whether it is a disease or not. This is one of those generally accepted social standards that may not be just or fair. In the practice of forensic pathology, cases of suicide are the ones that families are most likely to contest; sometimes these contests can become vicious and brutal. Nobody, not even close family members of the suicide victim, wants to be associated with someone who committed suicide.

Suicide is the end stage of a specific disease, like every other disease. Patients who attempt suicide or even commit suicide should be treated with sympathy or empathy like every other patient who is suffering from a fatal disease such as cancer. They should not be victimized and stigmatized, because the suicide may not, after all, be their fault, as in the case of Terry Long. It was not Terry's fault that he suffered from a disease of his brain that may have induced him to commit suicide.

Terry was indicted by federal authorities for some financial indiscretions in the terminal stages of his life and his disease. There exists a significant scientific probability that Terry's financial indiscretions, distorted psyche, failed businesses, and poor executive functioning may have been due to this underlying brain disease, caused by long-term repeated concussions of the brain. If Terry did not commit suicide, and if he had been tried for the criminal charges against him, I would have been willing to be the first expert witness to volunteer my services to defend a plea of insanity. No matter how far-fetched this possibility may seem, we must acknowledge this emerging reality. There is a significant scientific probability that if the hand of destiny had guided Terry Long on another path and he had not played football, he would have not committed suicide and would be alive today.

Since I examined and reported the findings on Terry Long's brain, I have developed a close relationship with his wife and family. I met his wife, Lynne, for coffee once and asked her to share vivid incidents about Terry at the peak of his disease. Several weeks later, she sent me the following e-mail:

There were over the years, irrational business
behaviors beginning in 1997 after we got married.
He opened TL's Inc. (ready-made salad producer for
Giant Eagle) with no experience in manufacturing.
From then, 1998, he contracted with Boggies Subs
to produce subs for Boggies (with no experience).
He financed both of these businesses from his own
personal finances. His business "risk" taking behavior seemed irrational, but you could never talk to
him about this. He saw it (his decision-making ability) as a "weakness" and often hid or tried to hide
his motivations/thought details of his business from
me. This often led to fights. . . . In 2000 both con-
tracts ended and from 2000-2002 he opened 5 new
businesses: CHIPS Inc. (food service manufacturing,
deli mainly), Handel's Ice Cream franchise, Deli/Hot
Meals Interstate business, Pizza Outlet business
and Value Added Foods, Inc. (a chicken processing
plant, again with no experience), all in rapid succes-
sion with no clear direction or product or customers.
He mortgaged and guaranteed millions of dollars of
loans with everything he had, which turned out to
be a fiasco. Terry had oscillating moods from kind to
violent without any warning. He was an easily like-
able guy and was able to develop friends very easily.
He would end up fist-fighting his new friends a day
or two later. His personality, fueled by his inability
to cope with his businesses, was always on either
extremes, but never with any warning of a shift or

any direct causal reason/basis for the change. This was the stranger side of Terry that always puzzled me.

Terry's autopsy findings have unraveled the puzzle of his behavior for Lynne. She is now at peace and hopes that no spouse of another NFL player will be placed in her dilemma again, for now we know better.

10

ANDRE "SPANKY" WATERS

I just want to take time to let you know how blessed I am to have you as my mother. . . . God placed you as my mother because He knew it was going to be successful. I needed a strong person, who could balance both love and fear . . . the love to get up every morning at 5:00 a.m. and go to work in the fields and come home at 6:00 p.m., wash clothes, hang them on the clothesline and still cook dinner. . . . They say God doesn't make mistakes and I have always believed that. Now I know for sure He doesn't make mistakes, because He blessed me with you. There isn't a day that goes by now that I don't thank God for blessing me with you as my mom. I love you today and everyday . . . especially today, my thoughts happily turn to you and my heart grows even more thankful, for all the years you gave me your best. . . . Happy Mother's Day.

Your son, *Andre M. Waters*

That is an excerpt of a letter from Andre "Spanky" Waters to his mother, Ms. Perry, which was written on the program booklet for Andre's funeral. Spanky was his mother's little boy. Out of her eleven children, five sons and six daughters, Andre, the ninth child, was her favorite. He was never a sickly child, and she had no problems with him. He was a smart and obedient boy who loved everybody. The name "Spanky" was given to him by his godmother when Andre was just a little child, and the name stuck with him even when he became a five-foot, eleven-inch-tall, two-hundred-pound NFL player. Andre and five of his siblings were raised single-handedly by their mother, who worked as a laborer in the cornfields in rural Florida and still did some housekeeping jobs on the side. Andre grew up very poor, and times were really rough.

The bond between mother and child prompted the teenage Andre to accompany his mom to the cornfields to work and make some money, which he wholeheartedly surrendered to his mom to place food on the family table. His mom hoped and prayed that her son would move ahead in life, go to school, become educated, and become somebody in life. He remained a calm individual with a big heart and loved helping and doing chores for other people. He was always eager to help his peers at school with schoolwork, was known to be jovial, made a jest of everything, had a great sense of humor, was not violent, and had no criminal history.

Andre Waters was born on March 10, 1962, in Belle Glade, Florida. As a child he played football on the streets with other kids and was known to dream and talk about the day he would become a professional football player. At a young age he became an active member of a Christian church and attended Sunday school. He began playing football in high school at the age of fifteen, and after he graduated from high school, football scouts identified young Andre as a budding football star. He was awarded a football scholarship to attend Cheney State University in Philadelphia, where he received a bachelor's degree in business administration. In his senior year at Cheney State, Andre became a member of the All-American Small College football team.

When he was hired by the Philadelphia Eagles in 1984, Andre Waters was an undrafted free agent out of Cheney State University. "It was by the grace of God that he [Andre] made it to the pros," his mother says. "As a young child he always believed he would be pro." He played for the Philadelphia Eagles from 1984 to 1993, and was a starting defensive back for eight years. In his rookie year in 1984 Andre returned a kickoff for an eighty-nine-yard game-winning touchdown. He moved on to play for the Arizona Cardinals in 1994 and 1995.

Andre's play was very aggressive. He was a vicious tackler and a brutal hitter. He became one of the NFL's hardest-hitting defenders, and his aggressive tackles resulted in the Andre Waters Rule, which prohibited defensive players from hitting quarterbacks below the waist while they were still in the pocket. He was nicknamed "Dirty Waters" by some. Andre was his team's leader in tackles for four seasons in 1986, 1987, 1988, and 1991. He had 910 tackles in his career and six consecutive 100-plus tackle campaigns from 1986 to 1991. He earned all-NFC honors in the 1991 NFL season.

Andre was a very determined athlete. Football was his escape from the abject poverty of his childhood. He was not going to live the way he did when he was a child. He worked extremely hard to stay in shape and jogged miles and miles every day. He was not known to have abused any steroids or other drugs.

When he became a rising football star, Andre did not forget his humble roots. He purchased a house and a car for his mother and gave her pocket money on a regular basis. He wanted his mother to stop working, but Ms. Perry did not want to stop working in the fields. He remained close and poured out his heart to his mother, making sure that he came home every Mother's Day and every Christmas to spend time with his mother and his family. When he was in the NFL, Andre was always delighted to have his mother come to the football field to watch him play. This was "until Mama told him she couldn't go watch football on Sundays 'cause Mama has to go to church."

Andre hid from Ms. Perry the injuries he sustained from playing football since he did not want her to worry about him. However, he always confided in his mother. He said, "Mama, when you hurt they even want you to play. They don't really care about you." He helped his brothers and sisters financially and would call and come home frequently. "He took care of everybody."

When he played for the Arizona Cardinals, Andre Waters admitted in an interview that he was knocked "woozy" while he played a game in high school early in the first quarter, when he hit the opposite team's tight end. After the hit, he was not fully aware of himself, but he continued playing, driven only by his instincts. Amazingly he did not know how he finished the first half. When he finally got himself together and fully realized where he was and what he was doing, the coaches were already going over halftime adjustments.

Many years after this incident, while Andre was playing in a game for the Philadelphia Eagles, he hit a running back helmet to helmet and he had a hard time getting up since he had lost his equilibrium. He got up slowly, but his coaches and team doctors did not realize he was hurt. They assumed that Andre always got up slowly after every hit. Andre ignored the many other concussions he sustained while he played in the NFL. The culture of the league was for players to condition themselves to play through concussions and musculoskeletal injuries, and ignore the pain until they could no longer play. After the fifteenth concussion while playing in the NFL, Andre lost count. He once said, "In most cases, nobody knew it but me. I just wouldn't say anything. I'd sniff some smelling salts, then go back in there" and play the game. For concussions, he said, "Feels strange, you don't know where you are. It seems like it gets darker around your eyes, like you're looking through some kind of telescope." According to the grapevine, Andre may have attempted suicide while he was still playing in the NFL.

After one of his many NFL games, Andre confided to his cousin Mike that he hit another player so hard that Andre himself got knocked out for a couple of seconds. Neither his teammates, his coaches, nor his team doctors realized it. He lay on the field for a brief period and regained consciousness only when another player bent over and called out his nickname, "Dre," several times. When Andre got up, he began to run in the direction of the opposing team's side until his teammates pulled him and turned him back in the direction of their team's side. Nobody on the field really bothered to take note of what had transpired with Andre, except Andre, and he kept it to himself.

Yet again, Andre Waters had a seizure after another game, while he was on the Philadelphia Eagles' team plane. The plane was being loaded with equipment at the Tampa International Airport. He was transported to a local Tampa hospital where he was admitted overnight. The seizure occurred on a Sunday night; Andre remained in the hospital until Monday afternoon, practiced on Wednesday, and played a game on Sunday.

When he left the NFL, Andre took a shot at teaching third- and fourth-graders. He did not like teaching, so he took up a football coaching career. He coached college football at Morgan State University, Baltimore, Maryland; Alabama State University, Montgomery, Alabama; St. Augustine College, Raleigh, North Carolina; Fort Valley State University, Macon, Georgia; and University of South Florida, Tampa, Florida. He worked on getting a coaching job in the NFL but was unsuccessful. He believed he had no mentor to help bring him into the NFL as a coach. Andre became extremely bitter about the NFL. He felt the NFL used players and dumped them when they no longer needed them.

Andre had filed for disability under the NFL retirement plan and was denied. He suffered one physical pain or another over his entire body from multiple blows sustained while playing football. He had fractured many bones in his fingers and toes and injured many joints. He suffered constant headaches and at some point began taking a narcotic analgesic, Percocet, in a desperate attempt to squelch his pain. Around 1995, Andre began to drink heavily, preferring brandy. He continued to drink heavily until 2000, when he started drinking only occasionally. He stopped drinking in 2004.

After his retirement from the NFL, Andre made some investments that did not work out. He and a friend opened a restaurant, which failed. He opened a pet grooming venture, which failed. With friends he invested money in several other businesses, which all came to naught. He made many bad judgments, spending money injudiciously and investing unwisely. People took advantage of his kind heart. He made bad judgments in his social life and social network as well. He kept bad company. A girlfriend once lied to him that her salary was six hundred thousand dollars per year. He believed her and began to spend heavily on her, later to find out that she made only thirty thousand dollars per year.

Mike, who was one of Andre's favorite cousins, lived with him from 1990 to 2002. Mike noticed around 1995–96 that Andre was becoming forgetful. While holding conversations Andre would suddenly forget what he was talking about and begin to use fillers like "emm, emm." He couldn't remember about conversations he had with people, including schedules, agreements, and plans. He began to frequently misplace his wallets, checkbooks, and keys, and he would search for them constantly. He was once known to have believed that his mother took his keys, when actually his keys were in his car. When he lived in a one-bedroom apartment in Raleigh, North Carolina, he would constantly lose things and forget about things. One day in 2006, when he lived in Tampa, Andre got lost while driving and he could not find his way home. He had to call a close female acquaintance to help him get home. It was said jokingly by his family that "Andre would lose his head if it was not on his body."

Andre was never married. He had girlfriends, but none of his girlfriends lived with him. He always had a cousin, a niece, or a nephew living with him, and he kept close ties with his family. Several times he got close to marrying some of his girlfriends, but something would always happen to prevent that. Apparently, the women broke his trust. According to the grapevine, Andre picked the wrong women, women who did not really care for him. He fathered three children with three different women, two sons and one daughter. He was involved in a drawn-out and emotional battle with his daughter's mother over child custody issues. Andre would say sometimes that he had everything in life except a good woman and a good wife.

Andre began living with one of his nieces, Terica, in an apartment in Raleigh in May 2003. He worked as the defensive coordinator for St. Augustine College, a liberal arts college. The team played in the CIAA (Central Intercollegiate Athletic Association) league. His niece was a student at St. Augustine. Andre resigned from this job in 2005. Apparently, he did not work well with his head coach, who ironically had been his head coach while Andre played college football at Cheney State University.

Terica had noticed something was going wrong with her beloved uncle in the summer of 2003. Andre was known to be an exuberant, outgoing, and sociable person who enjoyed family-centered activities and events such as cookouts and camping with his numerous nieces and nephews. However, Andre was progressively losing interest in these family activities and was beginning to dodge many of them. He would jump at every opportunity or provide any available reason to account for his absence from these family and social activities.

On Saturdays, Terica began to notice that Andre would lie in bed all day and not engage in any activities, especially when football season was over. He progressively developed a needy and dependent persona and became more private and seclusive. Beginning around 1997, Andre had begun to get upset and angry if people did not do what he wanted. This trait grew worse in 1998–99 and as the years went by.

During football seasons, Andre became excessively driven. He would stay awake all night at his office working on plays, watching game films, and breaking down plays. Early in the mornings he would come home, but as time went by, he would come home, take a shower, and go straight back to the office to continue working. He became more reclusive, withdrawn, and less driven when the football season was over. He was constantly restless. Even while he slept, he tossed, turned, and moved constantly. Sometimes he would go to bed late around 2:00 a.m. and wake up barely three hours later because he could not sleep.

He began to exhibit exaggerated responses to minor events and would blow things out of proportion. He seemingly overreacted to letdowns and disappointments and would get very angry and upset at times over issues that should not have upset anyone. Trivial things began to work him up emotionally, and he worried over everything. Little things bothered him, and he did not know how to let things go. An old office associate of his had once promised to send him something by mail and innocently forgot. Andre called her very irate and extremely upset, yelling at her on the phone and telling her never to speak to him again.

Andre exhibited fluctuations in mood. He would be upbeat and exuberant, then suddenly he would become sullen, a state that would last several days. As the years went by there were more sullen days. He became progressively isolated and did not want to be around a lot of people. One night Andre called a close friend crying, saying that he needed help and requesting that his friend help him. His friend reassured him that night and visited him in the morning to find Andre in an upbeat, happy mood, coming back from a barber's salon after a haircut.

Andre progressively lost his desire to throw parties, visit places of interest, attend shows, and socialize with his friends as he did while he was in the NFL. Ms. Perry observed obvious changes in Andre's behavior around 2003 when she noticed that when he visited her, he would lie around in the room all day and be very quiet. Andre mentioned suicide many times to family members and friends. In the final years of his life, he was constantly depressed and would always say to his cousin Mike, "I am very depressed." He told Mike that he wanted to kill himself, but Mike would always advise him and rationalize with him that there was no reason in the world that a guy like him should be depressed. On the occasion of one of Andre's suicidal ideations, he said to Mike, "I am gonna commit suicide. Are you gonna miss me?"

Andre was known to have attempted suicide many times after his retirement from the NFL. In one instance, he consumed prescription drugs. In two instances, he attempted to poison himself with carbon monoxide when he turned on the ignition of his car in a garage. On another instance, Andre had consumed a bottle of unspecified pills, but he did not die during the night. When he woke up in the morning, he said to his friend who was with him, "I guess I am still in the land of the living." In his final years he exhibited tearful episodes, and his suicidal ideations became more frequent. Minor life stressors induced him to verbalize thoughts of suicide to people who were close to him. Once Andre said to his niece, "What would you do if I die? Would you cry?" His niece said, "Yes." Andre responded, "You better not cry, because I will be in a better place."

Andre manifested a palpable fear of running out of money. He would complain about money one day and would come home the next day having gone on a shopping spree, buying all types of clothing and accessories like ties and cufflinks. People called him constantly asking for money, and he became less and less restrained and discreet with spending money. He was once known to have given a woman ten thousand dollars to purchase a home because she did not have money. He readily gave money to family members, friends, and acquaintances for a variety of reasons.

Andre Waters was painfully aware that there was something wrong with him, but he could not place a finger on it. He once said to a girlfriend, "I need help. Somebody help me." Mike noted that in Andre's final years he became a quiet guy who had the innocence and the heart of a five-year-old. He searched for answers by reading the Bible and religious books and thought there was something wrong with his relationship with God. He could not understand why he was so depressed even after he became a born-again Christian, professing and praying to God. Some of the students he coached remarked that Coach Andre always had his Bible with him.

Andre exhibited obvious paranoid ideations after his retirement from the NFL. He once told his mother that someone was against him and out to destroy him. He believed that people were not helping him to move up and that some of his superiors were not treating him well. He felt comfortable only at home and was not comfortable around a lot of people in social gatherings. When he visited nightclubs with Mike, he would not stay long inside the club and would rather go outside to watch his car since he was afraid someone was going to steal it. Andre and a friend of his joked sometimes that Andre was bipolar and should probably be on Prozac. However, on a more serious note, his friend advised him to consult a psychologist. He never did, although some of his family members believed that he probably began seeing a psychiatrist one to several years before he died. Andre did not mention or confirm this with his mother, nieces, or cousins.

Ms. Perry last saw her son on Mother's Day in November 2006. He had visited her and spent two to three nights. His mother prepared his favorite food for him. Andre loved chitlins. Whenever he came home his mother cooked chitlins for him with collard greens and sweet potatoes. Sometimes she cooked them and sent them to him in Tampa through a family member. The last thing Ms. Perry heard from her Spanky before he left home that final Mother's Day was, "Ma, I am ready to go now." Ms. Perry remembers his frequent calls, his visits, and favorite food. "I miss him. He was a loving son."

Andre Waters purchased a beautiful four-bedroom home in Tampa in 1987. He shot himself in the mouth shortly after 1:00 a.m. on November 20, 2006, in this home and was found dead by a longtime, close, female acquaintance. When she learned of her son's death, Ms. Perry wondered why Andre did what he did, especially when there was no history of depression or suicide in their extended family. Andre committed suicide just nine days after the end of the football season at Fort Valley State University, where he was defensive coordinator for the Division II team. His students, players, and colleagues, just like his mother, did not understand why Andre did what he did, since he was known to have a high energy level and exhibited an unsullied dedication to the game he cherished.

Following Andre's death in Tampa, Chris Nowinski, who had authored a book on concussions in football and who was personally interested in the subject, learned about the death and wondered if Andre's suicide may have been due to concussions. He contacted the medical examiner's office in Tampa and received a very cold shoulder. Chris was not a physician, so everybody pretended not to understand what he was talking about. Chris decided to seek me out because of the scientific papers I had published on the brain findings in two deceased NFL players with gridiron dementia.

I came home late some time in December 2006 on a cold winter day. I had just finished eating dinner and was watching the news when my home phone rang. A phone call at such a relaxing time of the day is not the least bit desirable. I was upset by the call, and I chose to ignore it. My wife, Prema, who happens to be a much calmer and more thoughtful person, rose from the couch and answered the call. She did not recognize who was calling, and she quietly asked me if I knew Chris Nowinski. His name rang a bell since he had interviewed me briefly for his book sometime prior. With curiosity, I took the phone and answered his call. That moment turned out to be one of the wisest of my life. I could have chosen to ignore the call, or I could have chosen to be nasty to Chris for calling me at such a bad time. But you should be nice to all persons, for you do not know when you encounter an angel. Chris turned out to be the angel who bore the prophetic message of gridiron dementia.

Chris informed me of Andre Waters's death and wondered if I could assist him with obtaining an informed family consent to perform tissue analysis on Andre's brain, to look for the tissue substrates of gridiron dementia or chronic traumatic encephalopathy. I asked him why he called me, and he said he thought I was the only person who could do exactly what he wanted. We set the ball rolling together; eventually we received a written consent from the Waters family, and we convinced the medical examiner's office in Tampa to send us archival sections of Andre's brain tissues. As a nonphysician, Chris accomplished all this almost single-handedly—no mean feat.

There are three groups of physicians: physicians who are conversant with current literature and know they are current with medical literature, physicians who are not conversant with current literature and know that they are not current with medical literature, and physicians who are not conversant with current literature and ironically do not know that they are not current with medical literature. The last group of physicians can be dangerous. Unfortunately, the physicians who performed the autopsy on Andre Waters were not aware of the association between brain injuries in general, repeated concussions in sports, and major depression and suicide. They were not conversant with this current literature and did not realize that they were not current with this medical literature. Consequently, they dissected Andre's brain in its fresh, mushy state and did not consider the reasonable probability of gridiron dementia being responsible for Andre's suicide. In fact, they would neither have talked with us nor cooperated with us if Chris had not worked so hard on securing an informed consent from the family ordering the physicians to release the tissues to us. One of the physicians even denied to the press that there was any association whatsoever between brain injury, dementia, and depression—even aside from the sports connection.

Thankfully, Andre Waters' family rose to the call and did the right thing by allowing us to perform tissue analysis on Andre's brain tissues. However, all that were saved in formalin from Andre's autopsied brain were five tiny pieces of brain tissue, which represented less than one-tenth of the entire brain and less than the surface area of an average adult palm. I called Chris and asked him to keep his fingers crossed. If the tissue analysis came back negative for grid-iron dementia, it would not necessarily mean that Andre did not have the disease since the volume of the submitted brain tissue was just too small. However, if the test came back positive, it would be most wonderful for our cause. And, wonderfully, the small brain sections revealed microscopic changes and abundant amounts of abnormal proteins that are typically found in the brains of eighty-plus-year-old individuals who have a certain type of dementia, changes similar to those found in the brains of boxers who suffer from dementia pugilistica or punch-drunk syndrome.

After I had called Chris to give him the paradoxical good news, what has happened since has been unbelievably amazing. On January 18, 2007, Alan Schwarz of the *New York Times* came up with a front-page story that read, "Pro Football: Expert Ties Ex-Player's Suicide to Brain Damage from Football." This article launched the issues of gridiron dementia, concussions in sports, and dementia and depression in athletes to a level neither Chris nor I would have ever imagined. Gridiron dementia became a national issue on many people's minds and in the media. Families and football players were emboldened to talk publicly about gridiron dementia, and it turned out that gridiron dementia was a hidden epidemic that had remained underrecognized. Many more NFL players may have suffered or are suffering from this disease in oblivion. It took three cases of autopsy-confirmed gridiron dementia to bring this disease to the limelight and public domain.

When asked about the strengths and weaknesses of her uncle, twenty-two-year-old Terica said this about Andre Waters:

> He was my superhero. I looked up to him. I was never concerned about his accomplishments. He did so much for me. I will miss his support. He was a very motivational person. About his weaknesses, I really hoped he could have gotten over his depression and problems, but now I know it was not his fault.

Truly speaking, now we know that it was neither Andre's weakness nor his fault that he did what he did or suffered how he suffered. Paradoxically, his strength on the football field led to his eventual weakness and demise.

EPILOGUE

11

WHY THIS BOOK WAS WRITTEN

W hy was this book written? So many reasons. There is no doubt that it may offend many people, while others will love it and embrace its message. Some people may be indifferent. The motivation behind the book should not be about our convictions and inclinations. It should rather be about seeking the underlying truth, for "you will learn the truth, and the truth will set you free." "And indeed everybody who does wrong hates the light and avoids it, for fear his actions should be exposed; but the man who lives by the truth comes out into the light so that it may be clearly seen that what he does is done in" truth. The objective of this book is not to criticize the NFL or American football and should not be deemed a captious judgment of the values and righteousness of the NFL.

The fundamental purpose of this book is to educate the wives, children, parents, brothers, and sisters of football players about this disease. Football players include players in youth recreational leagues and in junior high school, high school, college, and professional football. I hope this book will help them understand their loved ones better and become more tolerant and patient with these helpless victims of concussions. After all is said and done, their condition is not their fault.

Another purpose of this book is to educate fathers, mothers, uncles, aunties, grandparents, and others who want to decide whether to allow their preteenagers or teenagers to play football or not. In a free, democratic, and sophisticated society, every individual should be given the liberty to make such a decision. However, it has to be an informed and educated decision that should not be at whim. Like every endeavor in life, it is not just black or white. There is a wide gray area in the middle. Unfortunately most issues fall within gray zones, where individual preferences and convictions supersede.

The third purpose of this book is to sensitize sports trainers, coaches, and administrators to the dangers and delayed sequelae of concussions, especially repeated concussions sustained from playing football. Sports trainers, coaches, and administrators should take concussions more seriously, educating their players and collaborating with their medical staff to monitor and manage concussions more aggressively.

Another vital purpose of this book is to instigate a national and international discourse on the effects of concussions in sports. These effects have remained a long-ignored and hidden epidemic. We should not ignore this epidemic any longer, and we should not shy away from the discussion. The United States has the largest concentration of the best minds humanity can offer, having come from all parts of the world. The successes of the American economy have surpassed all imaginable objective predictions of macroeconomics in the nineteenth century—in fact, in the history of mankind. America is equipped with every wherewithal to study, understand, and overcome the threat of repeated concussions to the American way of life, for football is a vital component of the American psyche. The NFL, the guardian of the sport of football in the United States, has fallen short in its responsibility in preventing this disease. We should no longer wait for the NFL. As a modern society, we have to do something constructive because it is the right thing to do. People's lives are indeed at stake.

I must thank Chris Nowinski for his courage in writing his book *Head Games: Football's Concussion Crisis*. His book gave me the inspiration I desperately needed to write this book, and I encourage everyone to read Chris' book. It will provide us all with the historical and sociopolitical basis for the current concussion crisis that we face in American football.

Mike Webster, Terry Long, and Andre Waters have, through their deaths, taught us that gridiron dementia may manifest clinically, with the following elements of patient history, signs, and symptoms:

- **Previous history of amateur or professional play of football**

- Long latent period between first impact on the head in a game of football and manifestation of symptoms
- Progressive deterioration in social and cognitive functioning
- Loss of memory and memory disturbances
    Loss of language, incoherence
- Loss of executive functioning
    Dismal business/investment performance
    Dismal money management
    Deterioration in socioeconomic status
    Bankruptcy
- Paranoid ideations
- Social phobias
- Exaggerated responses to life stressors
    Bouts of anger, worry, and agitation over minor issues
- Rampant fluctuations in mood (highs and lows; happy and sullen)
- Breakdown of intimate and family relationships
    Spousal separation and divorces
    Spousal violence and abuse
- Increasing religiosity and quasi-spiritual insights
- Insomnia
- Hyperactivity, restlessness, high energy level, high performance drive levels
- Violent tendencies and criminal behavior
- Major depression
    Suicidal ideations and thoughts
    Suicide attempts/completed suicides
- Headaches, generalized body aches and pain

The composition of these signs and symptoms may well be known as Webster-Long-Waters syndrome. Simply put, if your husband, brother, uncle, nephew, cousin, or friend played football and begins to suffer or presently suffers from any combination of these symptoms, you may think of gridiron dementia and advise him to see a sports medicine physician. His symptoms may not just be one of those other routine psychiatric illnesses. He may need some special interventional treatment before it is too late. At least some types of experimental drugs have shown some promise in mammals and have reversed this disease. The same outcome is expected for higher mammals like us.

There is no doubt in my mind that in the near future we will discover more cases of gridiron dementia in retired football players and even in players of other contact sports. At the time of completion of this manuscript, I have received several calls from the close relatives and friends of retired football players who are suffering gridiron dementia in oblivion. I have actually examined the archival autopsy brain tissues of a fourth football player that revealed tissue evidence of gridiron dementia. His death was determined to be an accident by the coroner who performed his autopsy, but my investigation of his death and my interviews of his close friends and family members suggest that his death may have been a suicide. I have also received the autopsy brain tissues of another professional athlete who did not play football. He played another type of contact sport and had exhibited a syndromic psychiatric disease that was similar to the symptoms of gridiron dementia. With time the dementias of other types of contact sports will emerge, including wrestling dementia, ice hockey dementia, rugby dementia, and so on.

The players who have suffered and probably died from this disease want to be heard even from the land of the dead. Their spirits may be yearning to communicate with us to share their own sides of the story.

One day in summer 2007, I drove from Pittsburgh, Pennsylvania, to Morgantown, West Virginia, on a hot, dry, and clear day for a distance of about sixty miles, partly on Interstate 79 south. I had the formalin-fixed brain tissue of a deceased professional athlete in a plastic container secured on the back seat of my car. The family had granted me consent to examine the brain for tissue substrates of sports-induced dementia. I drove uneventfully for about one and one-half hours and arrived safely at the parking lot of the West Virginia University Health Center at about 1:20 p.m. I was eager and enthusiastic to process the brain tissue in the tissue laboratory. When I walked around the car to pick up the white plastic specimen container on the back seat, everything looked just fine. I proceeded to the tissue laboratory, processed the tissue over about three hours, and came back to my car in good spirits at about 5:00 p.m., only to realize that my right back tire was flat.

I called for road service assistance, and a technician came within thirty minutes to assist me with changing the tire. When we removed the tire, the technician remarked that the site of puncture looked peculiar and unusual. The tire, which was relatively new, was punctured at the side by a very tiny white piece of metal. He could not patch the puncture, so I had to buy new tires. I am not a superstitious person, so I did not even think about any possible link between the brain I carried in my car and the punctured tire. I drove back home upset that my tire was punctured but still glad that I had processed the brain.

I went to bed that evening at around 11:00. Again everything seemed fine. My pregnant wife went to bed two hours earlier. I joined her, and we slept peacefully just as we did most other nights in our young marriage. My wife woke up at around 5:30 a.m. to get ready for work since she worked from 7:00 a.m. to 7:00 p.m. three days a week as a registered nurse. When she got to the kitchen, she encountered something extremely unusual. The empty electric dishwasher was on and running. She was puzzled by what she saw, woke me up, and asked me if I had turned on the dishwasher. Of course, I did not turn on an empty dishwasher at 11:00 p.m., and even if I had, it would have shut off within six hours. I walked to the kitchen and switched the dishwasher off.

Then it clicked in my mind: first the brain tissue, then the punctured tire, and now the dishwasher. My wife was very upset and wanted to call our parish priest to bless the house and cast off any ghosts. I smiled and asked her not to worry about it. Not every ghost is evil. We have good ghosts. With her in the kitchen, I spoke out loud, addressing the thin air, and said, "Please, I promise you. I will do what I can do to help." I do not think he meant any harm. It may have just been his spirit wanting to convey his presence, to be acknowledged and reassured.

I have come to realize in life that all things may be possible, and you should never say never, and come what may, you should never be afraid. This professional player—just like his deceased colleagues who may have faced the same fate, who made the same sacrifices—may be reaching out to us in death to remind us of what we have long forgotten. We should not let him or any of them down.

AFTERWORD

I was born in a remote, rural village in eastern Nigeria during the somewhat primitive and tribal civil war between Nigeria and Biafra. The predominantly Igbo-speaking eastern Nigeria had seceded from the Republic of Nigeria to become a new country called Biafra. Nigeria had been granted independence from colonial rule by the British just six years earlier. The Igbos were fighting against the rest of Nigeria, which was predominantly made up of the Yoruba and Hausa tribes. The rationale for the war was primordial and based on ancient and seemingly petty tribal ideas, divisions, and convictions. Nevertheless, hundreds of thousands of Igbos were slaughtered and Biafra was run over by the Nigerian armed forces in about three years.

My pregnant mother and my family were refugees in a rural village in the jungles of Biafra, and my mother went into labor while the Nigerian Air Force carried out air raids, blasting scattered pockets and remnants of the decimated Biafran armed forces. My father was bedridden and lying critically ill in a wartime hospital bed with bandages over his entire body covering multiple shrapnel wounds. He had been a victim of an air raid several days prior when a bomb exploded close to his camp. My middle and vernacular name is "Ifeakandu," which means that life is the greatest gift of all. This name was given to me to memorialize the miraculous recovery of my father after I was born. Maybe I was the angel who bore his miracle to him. Who knows? Anyway, the war drew to its conclusion less than two years later. Biafra was vanquished. I survived the bombs, the hunger, and the tough life of a refugee infant. At least I did not suffer from severe malnutrition. I made it, just as I made it through so many hurdles and challenges in my later life, including the damaging effects of cultural shock and racism when I immigrated to the United States at the age of twenty-six.

I grew up an eccentric and extremely quiet kid. According to my older siblings, I was brilliant and adorable. I am the sixth of seven children, four boys and three girls. My father is a retired surface mining engineer and was the first in his entire extended family to receive a college education, although he was deserted in the earthen streets of his village by his mother, who had eloped with another man after the death of my grandfather. My father was only three years old. His father was a fisherman and had drowned in the village river while he was fishing. His death was suspected by the villagers to have been a homicide, but in those days in the jungles of rural Africa there were no forensic pathologists, and of course there were no forensic scientists who would have investigated a death that was apparently not witnessed.

The village missionary Catholic priest asked his cate-
chist to take my father in as house help, and helped him
achieve an elementary and secondary education. My father
served a British civil service administrator as a personal
assistant after secondary school. He was so loyal and hard
working that his boss secured him a scholarship to study
engineering in England. My mother was deprived of a high
school education when her father died suddenly, and she
had to stay home so that her brothers could go to school
since there was no money for her education. It was believed
that she would be married out to another family and cease
bearing her family name, so her education would benefit
her own family less than the education of her brothers who
would remain in the family and propagate the family name.
When she married my father, she attended a trade school to
learn tailoring. She became a self-employed seamstress and
designer and worked from home while she took care of her
children.

I started elementary school at the age of three. My older
brother, who was three years older than I, had to start at-
tending elementary school when he turned six. I was very
attached to him, and it was emotionally traumatic for me
whenever he left home to go to school. I cried so much that
my father approached the school principal and requested
that I be allowed to go to school with my brother for several days in order to smooth the transition of sibling sepa-
ration. The rest was history, for I went to school and even
outperformed the first-grade pupils who were at least three
years older than I. The principal retained me in school since
nobody had anything to lose. I maintained my academic
aptitude all through elementary and secondary schools and

entered medical school at the age of fifteen. I now regret it, for my academic pursuits robbed my childhood from me. I assumed adult roles too early.

I never wanted to become a physician. As a child I daydreamed about becoming a pilot who flew commercial jets on international routes. I dreamed about flying around the world from one big city to another and having in each city a beautiful girlfriend with whom I could spend blissful nights in condominiums whenever I flew into town. My parents stole my dreams away from me! I was a smart kid, and smart kids went to medical school. This was the prevailing social norm in the emerging elite of postcolonial Nigerian society in those days. I became a victim of that. Anyway, I was young, I was brainy, and I was an obedient child. I had to do what my parents wanted. I got into medical school, but in my fourth year of medical school I encountered a major developmental crisis. I became an emotional wreck. The busy and uptight life of a medical student was not my style. I wanted to be free. I wanted to fly around the world. The lives of medical students and even the lives of physicians generally were too regimented and boring for me. The same things over and over again, day after day. A medical career was not compatible with my inner self, with my God-given psyche.

Having been born in an air raid and having survived the hunger and malnutrition in a time of war, I was not the type to give up on medical school. Dropping out was not even an option. At this juncture I bargained and struck a deal with myself: I would finish medical school, but I would specialize in a field that was as far removed as possible from mainstream clinical medicine. By "mainstream clinical medicine," I meant specialties of medicine involving the care of living patients: family practice, psychiatry, surgery, pediatrics, and obstetrics/gynecology, for example. I had two options: radiology or pathology. I chose pathology. Yet, while specializing in pathology, I wanted a subspecialty of pathology that was even further removed from patient care. I chose forensic pathology.

What is forensic pathology? This takes us back to the etymology of the word *forensis*. From its remote Latin origin, this word has passed through hundreds of years of modifications and redefinitions. In modern-day parlance it means "after the fact." Since pathology is the study of the underlying causes of disease and the association of these causes with manifestations of disease, forensic pathology would refer to "after the fact of pathology." After disease comes what? Death. So forensic pathology is the study of death: its causes and its association with disease, trauma, and ill health. The old British term for the field was morbid anatomy or morbid pathology, but such a name is a little too direct for today's society.

There is nothing morbid about studying death, for death is a part of our lives. In living we die, and in dying we live. We can learn a lot from death, apply what we learn to our lives, and enhance the quality of our lives. Many epoch-making discoveries in the medical sciences have been made by studying death and have been applied to diverse human endeavors to improve the quality of human life.

While I was training to become a forensic pathologist, I realized that up to 60 to 80 percent of deaths involve the brain directly or indirectly, especially trauma-related deaths. I found the brain to be the most enigmatic and paradoxical organ in the body. It is one organ, yet it has hundreds of top-ographic component mini-organs that could function inde-pendently. Studying the brain appealed to me, so I applied for and enrolled in another two-year training fellowship in neuropathology. While I was studying neuropathology, I also realized that certain types of biomechanical loadings or transferences of kinetic energy would cause certain types of brain trauma. I became entranced by the patterns and spreads of brain trauma in the population, and I wanted to study them. Without a second thought, I enrolled in an-other two-year program to earn a master's in public health degree in epidemiology, the study of the spread and patterns of diseases in populations.

So here I am today with four board certifications—ana-tomic pathology, clinical pathology, forensic pathology, and neuropathology—along with a master's in public health de-gree in epidemiology, and I am now completing a master's in business administration degree from the Tepper School of Business at Carnegie Mellon University, one of the top twenty business schools in the world. You may ask why I chose to study business administration, for it has nothing whatsoever to do with my involvement with the brains of football players. But one thing I know: my added skill set in business administration enhanced my intellectual ability to manage and optimize the value propositions and utility functions of the findings in the brains of the football play-ers I have examined. You may call it a translational busi-ness management application, but it truly did help me get to where I am today regarding the subject of dementia in retired football players.

Really, though, my multifaceted background is not that unique. In the present age of information and knowledge economies, this type of intellectual preparation is becoming more and more the norm. A colleague of mine once said to me, innocently, "Bennet, why are you torturing yourself with all this education?" Quite simply, professionals are becoming more competitive and are beginning to acquire competencies in multiple specialties.

I started working as a combined forensic pathologist and neuropathologist in July 2002 under Dr. Cyril Wecht, one of the most brilliant, charming, and intuitive men I have met. He has contributed significantly to the circumstances that led to my studying the brains of NFL players. My present involvement in studying gridiron dementia comes directly from what I learned from Dr. Wecht and how he guided me in the very early phases of my career. Being a struggling young black African male in Pittsburgh in 2002 may have been challenging in certain aspects of professional life. Fortunately, Dr. Wecht did not only hire me to work for him; he supported me and even encouraged me to strive for my ideals while ignoring how people treated me and whatever people thought or said about me. Being an intellectually sophisticated man, Dr. Wecht provided a progressive and positive academic environment for me in the early days of my career, an environment that granted us access to the brains of NFL players and enabled us to identify for the first time the tissue substrates of gridiron dementia.

GLOSSARY

Abrasion. A scratch on the skin due to blunt force trauma.

Acute chemical meningitis. Inflammation of the coverings of the brain.

Alzheimer's disease. A common type of dementia in which brain cells and their nerve fibers are destroyed, impairing intelligence, cognition, memory, and behavior.

Amnesia. Loss of memory.

Amyloid plaque. Abnormal toxic forms of proteins that may accumulate in the brains of elderly people and in the brains of people suffering from certain types of dementia, including Alzheimer's disease.

Amyloid protein. A type of protein that is normally synthesized by cells in the body including brain cells.

Anabolic steroid. A group of hormones that supports tissue growth and normal functioning of cells in the body.

Anatomic pathology. A specialty of medicine that studies the structural basis of diseases.

Antibody. A specialized immune protein that binds to other types of proteins that are called antigens.

Asymptomatic. The absence of symptoms.

Autopsy. A systematic examination of a dead body to determine the presence or absence of diseases and injuries in order to determine the causes and circumstances of death.

Biomechanical engineer. A specialized engineer that applies the principles of engineering to the study, diagnosis, and treatment of diseases.

Biomechanical loading. The transference of kinetic energy to the body.

Biomechanics. The application of the laws and concepts of energy and forces to humans and animals.

Biomedical engineering. The application of the principles, concepts, and techniques of engineering in studying, diagnosing, and treating diseases.

Biopsy. A small amount of tissue removed from a person for study and disease diagnosis.

Bipolar. The fluctuation from one extreme to the other for example fluctuation of mood from elation to depression.

Brain. An organ that is part of the central nervous system and continuous with the spinal cord. It is enclosed within the skull and is the primary organ that controls and regulates all mental and physical bodily activities.

Cascade. A series of stages or events in which each stage derives from the previous stage and/or leads to the next stage.

Case report. A detailed report describing the causes, symptoms, signs, diagnosis, and treatment of a disease in a patient.

Case series. A collection of at least three case reports.

Cause of death. The underlying factor, event, or disease that initiates or instigates a terminal chain of events that finally culminates in death.

Cholesterol plaque. A semihardened buildup of a type of fat in blood vessels.

Chronic traumatic encephalopathy (CTE). A progressive degenerative disease (dementia) of the brain caused by traumatic injuries of the brain. The type of CTE found in boxers is called dementia pugilistica or punch-drunk syndrome. The type of CTE found in football players is called gridiron dementia or concussion-drunk syndrome.

Clinical pathology. A specialty of medicine that studies, identifies, and monitors causes of diseases using laboratory analyses of all types of body fluids.

Cognitive dysfunction. Abnormal intellectual functioning and loss of previously attained learned behavior and skills such as loss of memory, loss of language skills, loss of basic arithmetic skills, and loss of social skills.

Cognitive impairment. *See* cognitive dysfunction.

Cohort. A well-defined group of persons derived from the general population.

Concussion. Injury to the brain caused by the transfer of shearing forces to the brain.

Concussion-drunk syndrome. A degenerative disease of the brain caused by repeated concussions.

Concussions, three grades. Three different classifications of concussion based upon the severity of the symptoms and signs and the amounts of forces transferred to the brain.

Contributory factor. Factors that may alter the severity of a disease or injury, or factors that may accelerate death.

Contusion. A bruise caused by blunt force trauma.

Coroner. A public official who is responsible for investigating deaths especially violent deaths, suspicious deaths, and deaths with no obvious causes in order to determine the causes and circumstances of these deaths.

Dementia. A progressive degeneration of the brain with loss of brain cells and loss of normal functioning of the brain.

Dementia, football induced. A progressive degeneration of the brain (dementia) caused by repeated concussions of the brain sustained during the play of football.

Dementia pugilistica. A type of dementia caused by repeated punches to the head in amateur and professional boxers.

Depression. A type of illness distinguished by feelings of sadness, helplessness, worthlessness, and hopelessness.

Deviated joint. An improperly aligned joint.

Diffuse axonal injury. A type of injury to nerve fibers in the brain caused by shearing forces.

Emergency medicine physician. A specialized physician who treats patients in the emergency room when they require immediate medical attention and treatment.

Epidemiologist. A healthcare professional who studies the patterns and distributions of diseases in the general population.

Epidemiology. The study of the patterns and distributions of diseases in populations.

Etiology. The underlying cause of an entity like a disease.

Executive functioning. Higher intellectual abilities, such as self-regulation, prioritization of work, awareness of time, abstract reasoning, and logical analysis.

Explosive behavior. Hasty or impulsive bouts of anger, excitement, or aggression.

Forensic pathologist. A specialized physician who studies diseases and injuries as they relate to causes of death. A forensic pathologist performs autopsies to determine the causes and circumstances of death.

Formalin. A liquid chemical used to preserve human tissues and prevent them from decaying.

Fracture. Breakage of bones due to physical forces.

Gene allele. An alternative form of a gene, occupying a specific place on a chromosome.

Gridiron dementia. A type of dementia caused by repeated concussions sustained while playing football. Gridiron dementia may also be called concussion-drunk syndrome.

Intermittent explosive disorder. A disorder associated with hasty and impulsive acts of anger, excitement, or aggression, frequently due to poor impulse control.

Intracranial hemorrhage. Bleeding inside the cavity of the skull.

Laceration. A cut in the skin or soft tissues caused by a blunt force trauma.

Major depression. A severe form of depression. (*See* depression.)

Major depressive disorder. *See* major depression.

Manic-depressive disorder. A type of bipolar disorder whereby sufferers manifest unpredictable fluctuations in mood from periods of elation, excitement, and happiness to periods of depression and sadness.

Manner of death. The circumstances that surround death.

Mechanism of death. Events that link the underlying cause of death to the death.

Membrane. A layer of tissue that covers surfaces or separates regions of organs in animals and plants.

Mesothelioma. Cancer of the lining of the lungs.

Micrometer. A metric measurement equal to one millionth of a meter.

Microskeleton. Structural proteins that provide support and stability to nerve cells and nerve fibers.

Mild cognitive impairment. A disorder in which intellectual and mental capabilities are mildly impaired.

Millimeter. A metric measurement equal to one thousandth of a meter.

Molecular biologist. A specialized biologist who studies the structure and functions of genes and DNA.

Morbid anatomy/morbid pathology. The British term for the field of forensic pathology.

Nanometer. A metric measurement equal to one billionth of a meter.

Narcotic analgesic. A group of pain relievers that are derived from opium, for example, morphine.

Nerve cell. The cell of the nervous system that transmits, receives, and analyzes electrical signals.

Nerve fiber. A projection of a nerve cell that conducts electrical impulses to or from the nerve cell.

Neuritic thread. Abnormal nerve fibers containing abnormal tau protein, which is a type of microskeleton.

Neurofibrillary tangle. Abnormal structures in nerve cells formed by the accumulation of abnormal tau protein, which is a type of microskeleton.

Neurological. Relating to the nervous system.

Neurologist. A specialized physician who studies and treats disorders of the nervous system.

Neuropathologist. A specialized physician who studies tissues from the nervous system to derive diagnoses.

Neuropathology. A specialty of medicine that studies the structural and chemical basis of diseases of the nervous system.

Neuropsychiatric examination. A clinical examination of a patient, addressing mental, cognitive, intellectual, and behavioral problems.

Neuropsychiatric impairment. Abnormal functioning of the mental, cognitive, intellectual and behavioral domains of the brain.

Neuropsychological deficit. Impaired functioning of the mind in relation to understanding oneself and one's behavior.

Neuropsychologist. A medical specialist who studies the mind in relation to behavior.

Neuropsychology. A specialty of the life sciences that studies the functioning of the mind in relation to behavior.

Neuroradiological. Radiology of the central nervous system.

Neuroradiologist. A specialized physician who performs different types of radiological studies of the central nervous system, interprets radiological findings, and derives diagnoses.

Neurosurgeon. A specialized physician who treats diseases of the nervous system and performs surgeries on the central nervous system.

Neurotransmitters. Different types of proteins synthesized by nerve cells to enable certain types of interaction and communication between nerve cells.

Nonsteroidal analgesic. A pain medication that is not a derivative of steroids or opium.

Nuclei. Groups of similar nerve cells in different regions of the brain. Each group of nerve cells performs a specific function in the brain.

Organic brain disease. A general term that describes physical disorders or structural abnormalities that impair normal functioning of the brain.

Paranoia. Systematic delusions of persecution with irrational suspiciousness, fear, and distrustfulness of other individuals.

Paranoid ideation. Thoughts characterized by paranoia. (*See* paranoia.)

Parkinson's disease. A degenerative disease of the brain that affects nerve cells in the regions of the brain that control muscle movements and coordination.

Pathogenesis. The underlying causes and mechanisms of development of diseases.

Pathognomonic. A sign or symptom of a disease that is a defining feature for that disease.

Pathology. The specialty of medicine that studies the underlying causes and development of disease, the manifestations of disease, and the profiles and outcomes of disease.

Persona. The personality that a person projects in public.

Pharmacotherapy. The treatment of diseases with medications.

Postconcussion symptom. A symptom such as a headache or dizziness that occurs after a concussion.

Postconcussion syndrome. A compilation of symptoms and signs that may be present for a prolonged period of time following a concussion.

Pre-morbid. Before the onset of an event, especially a disease.

Psychiatric disorder. Abnormalities of the mind, thoughts, mood, and behavior.

Psychiatrist. A specialized physician who attends to and treats patients with mental, emotional, and behavioral disorders.

Punch-drunk syndrome. A type of degenerative disease of the brain or dementia seen in amateur and professional boxers caused by repeated blows to the head. It is also called dementia pugilistica.

Sensorium. Reception and interpretation of sensory stimuli by the brain.

Sentinel case. A new event or case indicating a larger underlying trend of events or cases that may have serious and adverse outcomes or consequences. Sentinel cases signal the need for immediate investigation and response.

Sequela. A complication, consequence, or secondary outcome of an event.

Shearing. Physical disruption or deformation of tissues by diffuse forces.

Sign. An objective physical manifestation of disease or trauma.

Sinus tract. A channel that connects a sac or space inside the body to the exterior.

Social phobia. Unjustified fear and anxiety about certain public places and gatherings, and social events.

Sports medicine physician. A specialized physician who attends to and treats athletes and players of all types of sports.

Subcellular level. At the level of the inside of a cell involving intricate and minute functioning of the cell; a scale or size smaller than cellular.

Subconcussion. Concussion of the brain that may not manifest with any symptoms or signs at the time of the concussion and is ignored by the sufferer.

Suicidal ideation. Thinking about killing oneself.

Suicide, completed. Successful, intentional or volitional, and premeditated act to kill oneself.

Symptom. A complaint or feeling of a patient that may be caused by a disease or trauma.

Syndromic psychiatric disease. A mental illness that has a characteristic group of symptoms and signs specific to that illness.

Synergism. A combined additive or multiplicative effect of two independent factors when the factors occur together. The exclusive individual effects of these factors are much less than their combined effects.

Tangle-only dementia. A type of dementia that occurs in the oldest of the old whose brains reveal many neurofibrillary tangles and neuritic threads.

Tau protein. A type of microskeleton that occurs normally in nerve cells and nerve fibers. May become abnormal in certain diseases and accumulate in nerve cells and nerve fibers to form neuritic threads and neurofibrillary tangles.

Topographic. Having to do with the structural relationships of different parts of the body and organs.

Utility function. The satisfaction of a consumer derived from the consumption of goods and services.

Webster-Long-Waters syndrome. The combination of possible symptoms and signs manifested by retired football players who are suffering from football induced dementia (gridiron dementia).

INDEX

About the Author

B ENNET OMALU was born in Nigeria, West Africa and immigrated to the United States in 1994. Dr. Omalu is a medical doctor with an MPH degree, as well as four board certifications in anatomic pathology, clinical pathology, forensic pathology, and neuropathology. He is currently completing a master's in business administration degree program at the Tepper School of Business, Carnegie Mellon University. Dr. Omalu performs autopsies and examines the brains of individuals who suffered brain injuries. He studies the relationship of brain injuries to death and the role played by brain injuries in the causation of death. He has published extensively in respected scientific journals and is a member of seventeen professional organizations. Dr. Omalu was the first person to identify gridiron dementia in the brains of NFL players. He has examined the brains of retired NFL players who suffered from dementia and major depression due to repeated concussions sustained from playing professional football.